Find videos demonstrating the most common surgical techniques in *Lateral Skull Base Surgery: The House Clinic Atlas* online at MediaCenter.thieme.com!

Simply visit MediaCenter.thieme.com **and, when prompted during the registration process, enter the scratch-off code below to get started today.**

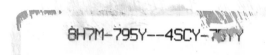

8H7M-795Y--4SCY-7?YY

This book cannot be returned once this panel has been scratched off.

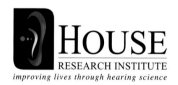

HOUSE
RESEARCH INSTITUTE
improving lives through hearing science

Videos available online:

1. Middle Fossa Approach
2. Retro-Sigmoid Craniotomy
3. Translabyrinthine Craniotomy
4. Transotic Approach
5. Combined Petrosal Approach
6. Temporal Bone Resection
7. Auditory Brainstem Implant
8. Blind Closure and CSF Leak Repair

Total length of videos: 1 hour

System requirements:

	WINDOWS	MAC	TABLET
Recommended Browser(s) **	Microsoft Internet Explorer 8.0 or later, Firefox 3.x	Firefox 3.x, Safari 4.x	HTML5 mobile browser. iPad — Safari. Opera Mobile — Tablet PCs preferred.
	** *all browsers should have JavaScript enabled*		
Flash Player Plug-in	Flash Player 9 or Higher* * *Mac users: ATI Rage 128 GPU does not support full-screen mode with hardware scaling*		Tablet PCs with Android OS support Flash 10.1
Minimum Hardware Configurations	Intel® Pentium® II 450 MHz, AMD Athlon™ 600 MHz or faster processor (or equivalent) 512 MB of RAM	PowerPC® G3 500 MHz or faster processor Intel Core™ Duo 1.33 GHz or faster processor 512MB of RAM	Minimum CPU powered at 800MHz 256MB DDR2 of RAM
Recommended for optimal usage experience	Monitor resolutions: • Normal (4:3) 1024×768 or Higher • Widescreen (16:9) 1280×720 or Higher • Widescreen (16:10) 1440×900 or Higher DSL/Cable internet connection at a minimum speed of 384.0 Kbps or faster WiFi 802.11 b/g preferred.		7-inch and 10-inch tablets on maximum resolution. WiFi connection is required.

Find us on Facebook *Connect with us on Facebook® for exclusive offers.*

Lateral Skull Base Surgery

The House Clinic Atlas

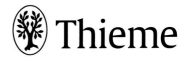

Lateral Skull Base Surgery
The House Clinic Atlas

Rick A. Friedman, MD, PhD
Associate of the House Clinic
Chief, Section on Genetic Disorders of the Ear
House Research Institute
Clinical Professor of Otolaryngology–Head and Neck Surgery
Keck School of Medicine
University of Southern California
Los Angeles, California

William H. Slattery III, MD
Associate of the House Clinic
Director, Clinical Studies Department
House Research Institute
Clinical Professor of Otolaryngology–Head and Neck Surgery
Keck School of Medicine
University of Southern California
Los Angeles, California

Derald E. Brackmann, MD
Associate of the House Clinic
Member of the Board of Directors of the House Research Institute
Clinical Professor of Otolaryngology–Head and Neck Surgery and Neurologic Surgery
Keck School of Medicine
University of Southern California
Los Angeles, California

Jose N. Fayad, MD
Associate of the House Clinic
Codirector, Department of Histopathology
House Research Institute
Chair, Otology Section
St. Vincent Medical Center
Clinical Professor of Otolaryngology–Head and Neck Surgery
Keck School of Medicine
University of Southern California
Los Angeles, California

Marc S. Schwartz, MD
Associate of the House Clinic
Chief, Division of Orthopedics Neurosurgery and Podiatry
St. Vincent Medical Center
Los Angeles, California

Illustrations by **Mark M. Miller**

Thieme
New York • Stuttgart

Thieme Medical Publishers, Inc.
333 Seventh Ave.
New York, NY 10001

Executive Editor: Timothy Hiscock
Managing Editor: J. Owen Zurhellen IV
Editorial Assistant: Elizabeth Berg
Editorial Director, Clinical Reference: Michael Wachinger
Production Editor: Barbara A. Chernow
International Production Director: Andreas Schabert
Senior Vice President, International Marketing and Sales: Cornelia Schulze
Vice President, Finance and Accounts: Sarah Vanderbilt
President: Brian D. Scanlan
Illustrator: Mark M. Miller
Compositor: Carol Pierson for Chernow Editorial Services, Inc.
Printer: Leo Paper Group

Library of Congress Cataloging-in-Publication Data

Lateral skull base surgery : the House Clinic atlas / editor-in-chief, Rick A. Friedman ; associate
editors, William H. Slattery III . . . [et al.].
      p. ; cm.
   Includes bibliographical references and index.
   ISBN 978-1-60406-764-4
   I. Friedman, Rick A. II. House Clinic
   [DNLM: 1. Skull Base—surgery—Atlases. 2. Skull Base Neoplasms—surgery—Atlases. WE 17]
   617.5'14—dc23   2011049356

Important note: Medical knowledge is ever-changing. As new research and clinical experience
broaden our knowledge, changes in treatment and drug therapy may be required. The authors
and editors of the material herein have consulted sources believed to be reliable in their efforts
to provide information that is complete and in accord with the standards accepted at the time
of publication. However, in view of the possibility of human error by the authors, editors, or
publisher of the work herein or changes in medical knowledge, neither the authors, editors, nor
publisher, nor any other party who has been involved in the preparation of this work, warrants
that the information contained herein is in every respect accurate or complete, and they are not
responsible for any errors or omissions or for the results obtained from use of such information.
Readers are encouraged to confirm the information contained herein with other sources. For
example, readers are advised to check the product information sheet included in the package
of each drug they plan to administer to be certain that the information contained in this
publication is accurate and that changes have not been made in the recommended dose or in
the contraindications for administration. This recommendation is of particular importance in
connection with new or infrequently used drugs.

Some of the product names, patents, and registered designs referred to in this book are in fact
registered trademarks or proprietary names even though specific reference to this fact is not
always made in the text. Therefore, the appearance of a name without designation as proprietary
is not to be construed as a representation by the publisher that it is in the public domain.

Printed in China

5 4 3 2 1

ISBN 978-1-60406-764-4
EISBN 978-1-58890-492-8

I dedicate this book to my wonderful sons, Andrew and Joshua,
for the love, joy, and wisdom they provide.
– R.A.F.

I dedicate this book to my family.
– W.H.S.

I dedicate this book to my family, who make it all worthwhile.
– D.E.B.

I dedicate this book to my many teachers, including Dr. Bernard Fraysse in
France, who guided my first steps in otology, and Dr. Antonio De la Cruz
and Dr. Fred H. Linthicum, Jr., who shepherded me through my research
fellowship and later my clinical fellowship in Los Angeles; to my associates
at the House Clinic; and to my family, especially my wife, Catherine, for her
unconditional support and sacrifices, my children, Nathalie and Daniel,
for all the joy they provide me, and my parents.
– J.N.F.

I dedicate this book to my family, teachers, and associates.
– M.S.S.

Contents

Accompanying Videos

Videos are available at MediaCenter.thieme.com

Foreword

◆ How It All Began

Back in 1936, during the last year of my residency at the Los Angeles County Hospital, I decided to limit my practice to otology. My brother Howard P. House was 15 years older than I and had an ENT practice that was 95% otology. The patients I saw in his practice impressed me because they were so grateful to have their ear problems properly managed. It seemed a much more gratifying practice than plastic and maxillofacial surgery, so I decided to become an otologist and to join Howard's practice.

During the last months of my residency, Howard had heard about Professor Wullstein in Würzburg, Germany, who had adapted to ear surgery a culposcope that had been designed by the Zeiss Company to examine the cervix for in situ cancer, so he took time off and traveled to Würzburg. This culposcope was revolutionary because it was balanced and could be easily moved to a new viewing angle and thus would stay in position without cumbersome screw tightening. Magnification could be changed without having to readjust the focal distance, and the light source was built-in, so that the operator looked through the cone of light; thus if it was lit, it could be viewed. While in Germany, Howard ordered one of these microscopes, the first to be sent to the United States, and my brother arranged for Professor Wullstein to visit the United States to lecture and demonstrate his work. He arrived in Los Angeles at about the same time as the microscope. We took the microscope to the morgue and Professor Wullstein spent an afternoon with us looking at temporal bone dissections through his scope. It is no exaggeration to say that I was stunned by what I saw. With the new microscope, I could now see all the details of the stapes, malleus, and incus, the blood vessels in the eardrum, and the mastoid air cells. (The first time looking through the microscope at the temporal bone reminded me of my experience when I was 12 and as a family we visited the Grand Canyon in Arizona. Standing at the canyon rim and looking at the grandeur of Creation I was overwhelmed. How did it happen? Why ask—it was the grandeur only God could create.)

Over the years I have never ceased to marvel at the beauty and grandeur of the temporal bone and hearing mechanism. I became and remained a microscope aficionado. For me, the era of microsurgery and my own future was born, but little did I realize then that due to this instrumentation my brother and I would be able to revolutionize otology, create a new field of neurotology, and found the House Clinic and House Research Institute.

◆ Teaching Others Microsurgery

Howard and I have always been dedicated to teaching otology; however, there was a problem in teaching microsurgery. During my first two years of practice, I did a large number of microsurgical ear operations with superior results. Because of this success, many doctors wanted to come to our Otologic Medical Group (OMG) to learn about microsurgery. The problem was that it was difficult to teach this surgery because the Zeiss Company's viewing tube required a visitor to stand by the surgeon and look through a viewing tube that had an image that was upside down and backward compared to the surgeon's own view. I resolved to determine if this viewer tube could be improved. Close by us in Hollywood were many optical companies connected with the film and aeronautical industries, so I looked for one to design a better viewing tube for the microscope.

In the first three interviews I had, I was asked how many of these could be expected to be sold if developed. My thinking was that there were perhaps 50 teaching institutions that could use them, so I said 50, maybe 75. I was immediately told the demand would not justify the effort. My fourth interview was with the Urban Optical Company. It was a small company that appeared to have only a handful of employees. I met with the owner, Jack Urban, in his small office; he listened carefully and thoughtfully to my problem and carefully examined the microscope head. He did not ask me about the demand, but simply said "Yes, I think I can do it." I was elated and asked how much he thought it would cost. I suppose he had sized me up as young and poor—he answered it would cost $500.00. I said I could pay that, and we started working together. Jack told me later he knew he could not do it for that amount of money, but at that time most of his work was defense related and he was no longer anxious to help blow up people. Jack and I developed a close working relationship and a loving respect for each other.

Jack often came to my operating room and learned firsthand about otologic microsurgery. Within six months he had a viewing tube that did not require the observer to bend over at an awkward angle and had the same view as the surgeon of the operative field. He adapted a small 16-mm gun camera used in fighter planes to film through the microscope during surgery. These cameras were small enough to avoid changing the balance of the microscope and interfering with the surgeon. In addition Jack adapted a sound system that could be recorded on the film. The films using these cameras that were subsequently made were invaluable in teaching otologic surgery. Later Jack was the first to adapt television cameras to the microscope. As is usual, the spectacular of today is the commonplace of tomorrow. Every operating room now has a microsurgery teaching facility.

◆ Training to Become a Neurotologist

The specialty of otolaryngology–head and neck surgery has greatly expanded since then. Today ENT residencies have faculty that are specialized in various areas of ENT. For this reason it would seem to me reasonable that the first year of ENT training should be spent rotating through the various aspects of ENT. At the end of this year, the resident can decide if she/he wishes to become a generalist in family practice groups doing ENT diagnosis, tonsillectomies, and some sinus surgery and be able to diagnose and refer patients with the problems presented in the chapters of this book for surgical management of lateral skull base lesions. During the remaining time of the residency, those striving to become neurotologists should spend 3 hours each week in temporal bone dissection. They need to be able to mentally visualize the temporal bone anatomy in 3D when viewed from the post auricular, superior, and anterior perspectives. This way, during surgery, wherever you are in the temporal bone you know the structures that are adjacent. It usually takes several months to achieve this perspective. During this time they should observe videos of skull base surgery, such as those that accompany this book, and assist with cases during surgery. Finally they should perform the various procedures on frozen heads that have preferably not been embalmed. In addition patient evaluation and postoperative follow-up clinics should be included in the weekly schedule.

◆ The Legacy Continues

The House Clinic and the House Research Institute that my brother and I founded have grown tremendously over the years. The current staff at the House Clinic includes ten surgeons who are among the best and brightest in the world. Medical students, residents, fellows, and practitioners continue to come to the Clinic for state-of-the-art training in the latest technology and techniques. I want to congratulate Rick A. Friedman, William H. Slattery III, Derald E. Brackmann, Jose N. Fayad, and Marc S. Schwartz for this edifying book. With a legacy of excellence started over 75 years ago, it is extraordinarily exciting to see the House Clinic continuing to set the standard for excellence in patient care and education.

William F. House, MD, DDS
Aurora, Oregon

Preface

This atlas of lateral skull base surgery is the culmination of hundreds of physician-years of combined experience from our center. Modern neurotology (lateral skull base surgery) was born in Los Angeles with the combined brilliance and thoughtful collaboration of Howard P. House, William F. House, and William E. Hitselberger. Their fearless innovation led to a dramatic decrease in the mortality and morbidity of surgery for tumors of the skull base, most notably vestibular schwannoma. They ushered in an era that went beyond lifesaving surgery to functional facial motor and hearing preservation.

In this book, the authors of the next generation share their continued experience with the surgical management of skull base lesions. Although the treatment strategies for tumors of the skull base are in constant evolution, when surgery is indicated, staying true to the methods of our predecessors, we continue to provide outstanding care for our patients.

Acknowledgments

The House Clinic of Los Angeles, California, is known to have one of the largest fonts of experience in the world managing difficult skull base lesions. It was the unique vision, innovation, and collaboration of Howard P. House, William F. House, and William E. Hitselberger, who laid the groundwork for modern neurotology. The five editors of this book acknowledge the efforts of those three, which have set the gold standard for the care of this patient population.

We thank our book's contributors for their efforts, and we thank artist Mark M. Miller for his richly detailed drawings. We thank the Anspach Effort, Inc. of Palm Beach Gardens, Florida, for their kind assistance to the art program.

Contributors

Marc K. Bassim, MD
Assistant Professor of Otolaryngology–
    Head and Neck Surgery
American University of Beirut Medical
    Center
Beirut, Lebanon

Derald E. Brackmann, MD
Associate of the House Clinic
Member of the Board of Directors
    of the House Research Institute
Clinical Professor of Otolaryngology–
    Head and Neck Surgery and
    Neurologic Surgery
Keck School of Medicine
University of Southern California
Los Angeles, California

Robert D. Cullen, MD
Otologic Center
Kansas City, Missouri

Antonio De la Cruz, MD‡
Associate of the House Clinic
Director of Education
House Research Institute
Clinical Professor of Otolaryngology–
    Head and Neck Surgery
Keck School of Medicine
University of Southern California
Los Angeles, California
[‡Deceased]

Jose N. Fayad, MD
Associate of the House Clinic
Codirector, Department of
    Histopathology
House Research Institute
Chair, Otology Section
St. Vincent Medical Center
Clinical Professor of Otolaryngology–
    Head and Neck Surgery
Keck School of Medicine
University of Southern California
Los Angeles, California

Rick A. Friedman, MD, PhD
Associate of the House Clinic
Chief, Section on Genetic Disorders
    of the Ear
House Research Institute
Clinical Professor of Otolaryngology–
    Head and Neck Surgery
Keck School of Medicine
University of Southern California
Los Angeles, California

L. Fernando Gonzalez, MD
Assistant Professor of
    Neurosurgery
Jefferson Medical College
Thomas Jefferson University
Philadelphia, Pennsylvania

William E. Hitselberger, MD
Neurosurgeon
Los Angeles, California

John W. House, MD
President
House Research Institute
Clinical Professor of Otolaryngology–
    Head and Neck Surgery
Keck School of Medicine
University of Southern California
Los Angeles, California

J. Walter Kutz, Jr., MD
Assistant Professor of Otolaryngology–
    Head and Neck Surgery
University of Texas Southwestern
    Medical Center
Dallas, Texas

Gregory P. Lekovic, MD
Staff Neurosurgeon of the House
    Clinic
Adjunct Scientist of the House
    Research Institute
Los Angeles, California

James Lin, MD
Assistant Professor of Ontolaryngology
Kansas University Medical Center
Kansas City, Kansas

William M. Luxford, MD
Associate of the House Clinic
Clinical Professor of Otolaryngology
Keck School of Medicine
University of Southern California
Los Angeles, California

Felipe Santos, MD
Instructor of Otology and Laryngology
Massachusetts Eye and Ear Infirmary
Harvard Medical School
Boston, Massachusetts

Marc S. Schwartz, MD
Associate of the House Clinic
Chief, Division of Orthopedics
    Neurosurgery and Podiatry
St. Vincent Medical Center
Los Angeles, California

Maroun T. Semaan, MD
Assistant Professor of Otolaryngology–
    Head and Neck Surgery
University Hospital Ear Nose and Throat
    Institute
Case Medical Center, Case Western
    Reserve University
Cleveland, Ohio

William H. Slattery, MD
Associate of the House Clinic
Director, Clinical Studies Department
House Research Institute
Clinical Professor of Otolaryngology–
    Head and Neck Surgery
Keck School of Medicine
University of Southern California
Los Angeles, California

Karen Borne Teufert, MD
House Research Institute
Los Angeles, California

Eric P. Wilkinson, MD, FACS
Associate of the House Clinic
Adjunct Research Scientist
House Research Institute
Clinical Assistant Professor of
    Otolaryngology–Head and Neck
    Surgery
Keck School of Medicine
University of Southern California
Los Angeles, California

1

Orbitozygomatic Craniotomy

Gregory P. Lekovic, L. Fernando Gonzalez,
Felipe Santos, and Marc S. Schwartz

The guiding principle of skull base surgery is the avoidance of brain retraction by the removal of additional bone. The orbitozygomatic craniotomy may augment exposure under the frontal lobe, through the sylvian fissure, along the tip of the temporal lobe, and in other locations. The initially described approach includes removal of the superior and lateral orbital rim as well as the zygomatic arch. This approach may be tailored to specific pathology as well. This chapter describes the standard orbitozygomatic craniotomy as well as several variations that may be used to either reduce or extend dissection as indicated for different situations.

The main advantages of the orbitozygomatic approach are (1) the supraorbital rim is removed from the surgeon's line of sight, facilitating an upward and oblique view to the interpeduncular fossa and third ventricle; and (2) the temporalis muscle is retracted laterally and inferiorly, instead of anteriorly, by removing the arch of the zygoma, thus giving the surgeon a much wider corridor within which to approach deep-seated lesions for which the alternative would be a traditional subtemporal approach. Finally, the extent of bone removal minimizes brain retraction and makes the orbitozygomatic approach ideal for extradural approaches to the cavernous sinus and anterior petrous apex.

◆ Surgical Anatomy

The frontal branch of the facial nerve leaves the pes anserinus in the parotid, lies deep to the temporoparietal fascia, and may be injured during scalp dissection. The temporoparietal fascia is in continuity with the galea superiorly and the superficial musculoaponeurotic system (SMAS) inferiorly. There is an avascular loose areolar tissue layer between this and the underlying deep temporal fascia that is in continuity with the subgaleal plane. Superiorly, the deep temporalis fascia is a single sheet that splits into two layers (superficial layer and deep layer of the deep temporal fascia) enveloping the superficial temporal fat pad. In addition, care should be taken to preserve, whenever possible, the superficial temporal artery. Though in our experience vascular compromise of the flap has not been an issue when this artery is sacrificed during exposure, its preservation may be critical in those rare instances where a low-flow extracranial to intracranial bypass is needed.

The medial extent of the orbitozygomatic craniotomy is usually demarcated by the supraorbital notch, through which travel the supraorbital nerve and an associated vascular bundle. When encased completely in bone or more laterally situated than usual, it can be easily mobilized with an osteotome if needed. The inferior extent of the orbitozygomatic exposure is limited by the zygomaticofacial foramen. The posterior border of the bony exposure runs along a line connecting the supraorbital to infraorbital fissures. The key landmark for the successful completion of the orbitozygomatic osteotomies is this latter completely extracranial fissure in the inferolateral wall of the orbit. It can be palpated from within the orbit with a Penfield No. 4 dissector, and is the starting point for the reciprocating saw cut through the malar eminence. Similarly, it is the point to which the reciprocating cuts through the sphenoid bone from the superior orbital fissure connect. Hence, at the completion of the "full" orbitozygomatic (OZ) osteotomy, the surgeon removes the roof and lateral wall of the orbit en bloc. This facilitates orbital reconstruction and reduces the risk of enophthalmos postoperatively.

◆ Preoperative Workup

Gadolinium-enhanced magnetic resonance imaging is essential for planning for all tumors of the skull base; for intraorbital tumors and for those in the petrous apex and or clivus, fat suppression should be obtained as well. For paraclinoid aneurysms of the internal carotid artery, computed tomography angiography (CTA) is very helpful in determining the relationship of the aneurysm origin to the optic strut; this in turn helps differentiate cavernous sinus aneurysms from those that risk rupture into the subarachnoid space. In fact, digital subtraction angiography can usually be avoided for most aneurysms; high-resolution preoperative CTA or magnetic resonance angiography (MRA) is sufficient for surgical planning.

◆ Surgical Technique

Monitoring

We routinely monitor somatosensory evoked potentials intraoperatively; depending on the nature of the pathology, motor evoked potentials or electrocorticography may be indicated as well. In our experience motor evoked potentials require total intravenous anesthesia, as inhalational anaesthetics cause degradation of the motor response over time.

Anesthetic Considerations

Serial compression devices are placed on all patients, and all patients receive perioperative antibiotics. We prefer cefuroxime 1.5 g IV. Intravenous mannitol up to 1 g/kg may be given to facilitate brain relaxation. As mentioned above, muscle relaxants are avoided or eliminated to optimize electrophysiologic monitoring. For vascular lesions, anesthesiology should be prepared to administer barbiturates for burst suppression, and to induce hypotension if needed.

Variations

Full Orbitozygomatic Craniotomy

The patient is rigidly fixated in a Mayfield head holder and positioned slightly vertex down with the head rotated to the contralateral side, so that the ipsilateral malar eminence is at the top of the operative field. A fingerbreadth of hair along the planned incision is clipped and the skin infiltrated with local anesthetic. The scalp incision extends from the root of the zygoma, just anterior to the tragus, to past midline, at the level of the contralateral midpupillary line, just behind the hairline (**Fig. 1.1**). The pericranium should be elevated separately in case the frontal sinus is violated during the orbital osteotomies.

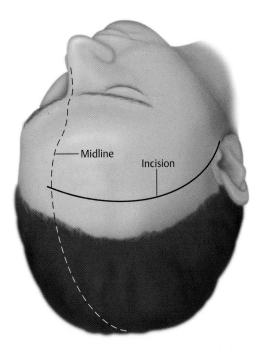

Fig. 1.1 Frontotemporal scalp incision just behind the hairline. The anterior limb of the incision is typically brought across midline.

Injury to the frontal branch of the facial nerve can be avoided either by performing a subfascial dissection of the temporalis fascia, or through an interfascial dissection. This latter approach is more time-consuming. Practically speaking, the nerve travels in the fat pad between the superficial and deep layers of the temporalis fascia within a fingerbreadth of the supraorbital rim; hence, injury to the nerve can reliably be avoided by performing a subfascial dissection from this point forward (approximately 3 cm behind the supraorbital rim at the temporal line).

Next, the supraorbital rim, frontozygomatic process, and malar eminence are exposed by elevating the frontal pericranium and temporalis fascia with a sharp-edged periosteal elevator. The root of the zygoma can usually be palpated, and the superficial investment of the temporalis fascia on the temporal zygomatic arch dissected free (**Fig. 1.2**).

Next, the periorbita is elevated from the roof of the orbit with a Penfield No. 1 elevator. Thin cottonoids or Telfa strips may be used both to facilitate the dissection and protect the periorbita from tearing (**Fig. 1.3**). It is often impossible to elevate the periorbita without tearing it. This may result in the periorbital fat herniating through the opening and obscuring the surgeon's line of sight, in which case the fat can be shrunk with bipolar coagulation and small rents in the periorbita tacked closed with 4–0 Nurolon suture.

The temporalis muscle is then split and its deep periosteal attachment elevated from inferior to superior, staying in the direction of the fibers of the muscle. We prefer to split the muscle sharply and obtain hemostasis with bipolar electrocautery, rather than incising the muscle with the Bovie, to minimize temporalis atrophy (**Fig. 1.4**). The temporalis muscle is then reflected anteriorly and secured with fishhooks. The pterion is identified, and bur holes placed on either side of the greater wing of the sphenoid. A standard, kidney-bean–shaped pterional flap is then elevated. Although for the "two-piece" OZ craniotomy it is not critical for a bur hole to be placed at the true McCarty "keyhole," positioning this flap as close to the floor of the anterior fossa

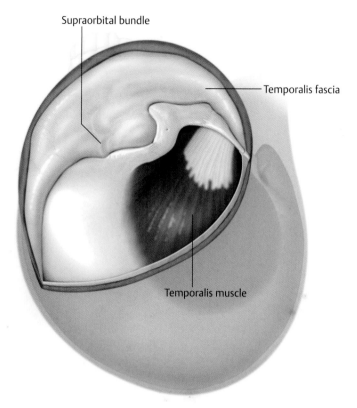

Fig. 1.2 Reflected scalp showing exposure of the orbital rim and zygoma. Care is taken to expose medial to the supraorbital bundle. The root of the zygoma is exposed circumferentially.

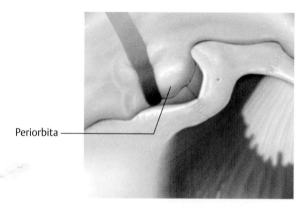

Fig. 1.3 Elevation of periorbita using a sharp-edged instrument such as a Penfield No. 1 elevator. Cottonoid or Telfa strips may be useful in protecting orbital contents, which tend to herniated through the very thin and typically adherent periorbita.

(i.e., as close to the orbital roof) as possible and incorporating as much of the greater wing of the sphenoid as possible greatly facilitates visualization of the subsequent orbitozygomatic osteotomies (**Fig. 1.5**).

Attention then is turned back to preparation for the orbitozygomatic osteotomies. The temporalis muscle is released from the fishhooks and placed back over the crani-

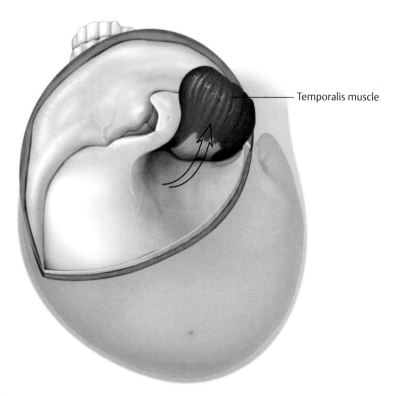
Temporalis muscle

Fig. 1.4 Elevation of temporalis muscle. The muscle must be completely lifted from the pterional region down to the level of the zygomatic arch.

otomy defect. At the completion of these maneuvers, the entire zygomatic arch and malar eminence should be exposed. For the traditional, "full" orbitozygomatic approach, a reciprocating saw is used to make six osteotomies. The first osteotomy is made at the base of the zygoma by placing the saw on the zygomatic root just above the temporalis muscle. Prior to making the cut, a low-profile fixation plate is fixed to the anterior portion of the arch and the posterior hole for the plate is drilled; this maneuver ensures a good reapproximation of the zygoma on closing. The cut through the zygoma is oriented obliquely and anteriorly so that the two edges of the bone overlap. Care must be taken not to violate the capsule of the temporomandibular joint. The second cut begins just inferior to the temporal process of the zygomatic bone where it adjoins the malar eminence and proceeds anteriorly at an oblique angle; care must be taken to avoid the zygomaticofacial foramen. The third osteotomy extends from the inferior orbital fissure from within the orbit through the orbital surface of the temporal bone to connect with this second cut. The inferior orbital fissure can be palpated with a Penfield No. 4 dissector, and this is where the tip of the reciprocating saw is placed, oriented outward toward the previous cut in the malar eminence at an angle so that when joined they make an inverted V.

The fourth cut extends through the orbital surface of the frontal bone posteriorly as a continuation of the medial exposure of the pterional craniotomy. This cut is often described as extending all the way back to the superior orbital fissure, though in practice it instead curves gently back approximately 3 cm toward the lateral wing of the same. After completing the fourth cut, we recommend pre-fitting microplates at the lateral and superior orbital rim. Plates are aligned and all screws temporarily driven at this point. This will allow for proper realignment during craniofacial reconstruction. The fifth osteotomy extends posteriorly from the inferior orbital fissure across the greater wing of the sphenoid bone and through the posterior orbit. The final

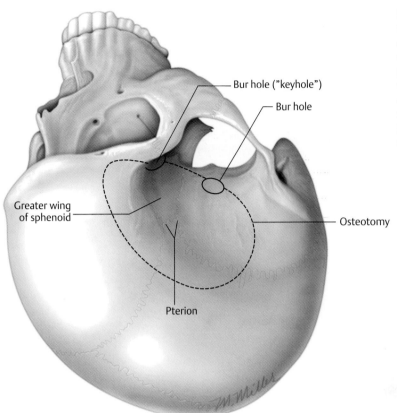

Fig. 1.5 Completion of craniotomy. **(A)** Extent of a first-stage craniotomy in the standard frontotemporal location. **(B)** Surgeon's view showing osteotomies necessary for removal of orbitozygomatic flap. **(C)** Frontal view of the same. The cuts are made is this order: 1, root of the zygoma; 2, inferior zygoma; 3, lateral orbit; 4, superior orbit; 5, inferior orbital fissure to sphenoid wing; 6, sphenoid wing to superior orbit.

Bur hole ("keyhole")

Bur hole

Greater wing
of sphenoid

Osteotomy

Pterion

A

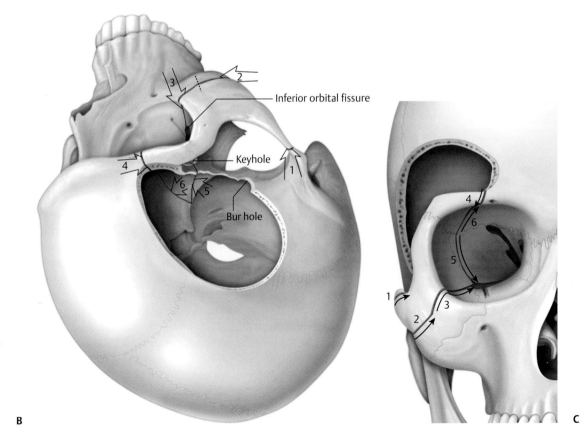

Inferior orbital fissure

Keyhole

Bur hole

B

C

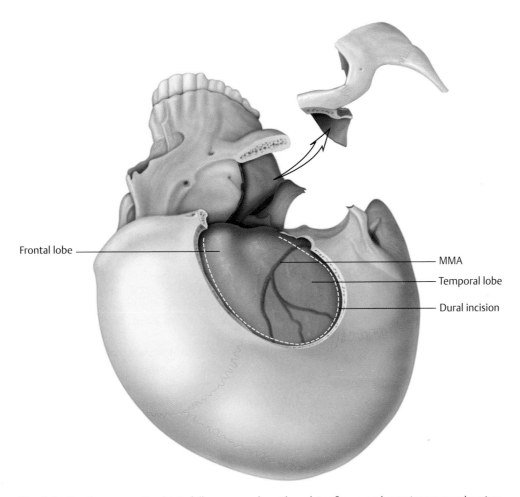

Frontal lobe

MMA

Temporal lobe

Dural incision

Fig. 1.6 Dural exposure. To obtain full exposure along the sylvian fissure and anterior temporal region, the remainder of the greater sphenoid wing is resected, and the meningo-orbital artery and vein at the lateral end of the superior orbital fissure are divided. MMA, middle meningeal artery.

(sixth) osteotomy extends from the superior orbital fissure (SOF), or from the most inferior and lateral portion of the fourth cut proximal to the SOF, laterally to meet the cut in the sphenoid bone through the lateral orbit from the inferior orbital fissure; that is, it connects the fourth and fifth osteotomies. A rongeur can be used to remove the residual bony island of the greater wing of the sphenoid until the dural fold of the SOF is identified (**Fig. 1.6**).

The meningo-orbital artery and associated vein exit the SOF along its lateral aspect and penetrate the dura. This vascular bundle should be coagulated and cut to mobilize the dura of the temporal pole. Failure to recognize this fold of dura and coagulate the artery within it will frustrate the surgeon's attempts to approach the cavernous sinus and anterior clinoid process.

For lesions located intradurally, the dura is opened from the medial superior orbital margin to the temporal tip in a semilunar fashion. Dural tack-up sutures are placed anteroinferiorly, which permits downward retraction of the globe. They should be placed as deep toward the orbital apex as possible and anchored around the secure fishhooks. The operating microscope is then brought into the field, and standard transsylvian or subtemporal approaches performed as dictated by individual pathology.

Modified Orbitozygomatic Craniotomy

Some situations call for orbital osteotomy to maximize exposure in the subfrontal plane but do not require extended lateral exposure. In these cases, the zygomatic arch can be left intact. In practice, most anterior circulation aneurysms can be approached with either of the following modifications to the traditional OZ osteotomy. Because the mini-supraorbital craniotomy provides limited lateral exposure, its use for lateral skull base lesions is limited and will not be discussed in detail.

The authors prefer to elevate the modified orbitozygomatic craniotomy as a single flap; we believe this is cosmetically preferable for the patient, as there is less need for fixation plates over the supraorbital rim, and it can be done without sacrificing any needed exposure. One-piece bony removal may not be appropriate, however, with some tumors that may cause bony changes in the orbital roof and optic canal. In these cases, there may be added risk to the optic nerve with elevation of the craniotomy in a single flap, and the orbital rim can be removed under direct vision after standard frontal craniotomy.

Preoperative considerations and the initial patient positioning are much the same for the modified OZ craniotomy as for the traditional approach. An interfascial or subfascial dissection is not necessary, however, as the temporalis muscle will be reflected anteriorly with its fascia. Rather, a cuff of temporalis fascia is left along its attachment to facilitate reapproximation.

In contrast with the "full" approach, proper placement of a "keyhole" bur hole exposing the dura of the anterior fossa and periorbita is crucial to successful completion of the modified orbitozygomatic craniotomy. This bur hole is important for two reasons: (1) the roof of the orbit is identified, which is particularly useful if the orbital roof is thick and difficult to fracture; and (2) it allows the surgeon to extend the cut laterally through the orbital wall past the frontozygomatic suture. After this bur hole is placed, a craniotome is used to prepare the pterional portion of the craniotomy, as is the case with the full OZ craniotomy, as the craniotomy is extended as inferiorly as possible, just lateral to the supraorbital notch. Instead of the six osteotomies of the full OZ craniotomy, in the modified OZ craniotomy only three osteotomies need to be performed. The first of these is performed with a reciprocating saw through the frontal process of the zygoma just lateral to the frontozygomatic suture. The second cut is a continuation of the craniotome cut in the sagittal plane through the roof of the orbit just lateral to the supraorbital notch. The dura can be elevated off the roof of the orbit with a small Penfield dissector and a cottonoid patty placed on the surface of the dura to protect it from the reciprocating saw, similar to the dissection of the periorbita. In practice, this second osteotomy never extends as deeply posterior as is possible with the two-piece or "full" OZ variations. We prefer to make the third osteotomy with a small hand-held osteotome, through the roof of the orbit exposed in the keyhole oriented medially toward the second cut. Alternatively, the roof of the orbit can simply be fractured free.

Extended Orbitozygomatic: Trans–Cavernous Sinus Approach

The orbitozygomatic approach can be extended via entry into the cavernous sinus for exposure of cranial nerves (CNs) III, IV, and VI. In conjunction with posterior clinoidectomy, the cavernous sinus can be traversed for enhanced exposure of posterior fossa structures including the contents of the basal cisterns, superior clivus, and the mid-basilar artery and its branches. The second and third divisions of the trigeminal nerve are readily exposed with dissection of the dura propria from the lateral wall of the cavernous sinus, without necessitating further bony removal.

The first step in exposure of the cavernous sinus is the development of the plane between the anterior temporal pole and cavernous sinus, which is necessary to allow for retraction of the temporal lobe. Dividing the meningo-orbital vascular bundle and dural fold as described above in the description of the traditional OZ craniotomy allows the surgeon to develop the plane between the two outer leaflets of the cavernous sinus dura. The dura propria, or dura of the anterior pole of the temporal lobe, can thus be separated from the inner dural leaflet investing the superior orbital fissure and cavernous sinus proper. This dissection is best performed sharply, and is limited by V3 posteriorly and the tentorium medially. This maneuver by itself provides excellent distal exposure of the trigeminal nerve, foramen rotundum, and ovale, and can be combined very effectively with an extended middle fossa approach for schwannomas of the trigeminal nerve.

The anterior clinoid process is the medial extension of the sphenoid wing, and forms a barrier to visualization of the proximal carotid artery and medial contents of the cavernous sinus. Anterior clinoidectomy may be performed either extradurally or intradurally; we prefer the extradural approach. As an isolated maneuver, anterior clinoidectomy provides wide intradural exposure of the basal cisterns and optic nerve, the infraclinoid portion of the internal carotid artery, and the cisternal portion of the oculomotor nerve. Mobilization of the internal carotid artery with dissection of the proximal and distal dural rings further exposes the infraclinoid carotid artery, and allows access to the medial cavernous sinus and carotid siphon. Bone removal is carried to the optic canal, which is widely decompressed. The anatomy of the anterior clinoid is variable, but after decompression of the posterior orbit and the optic canal, the remaining point of bony attachment is the optic strut, which runs between the optic nerve and the internal carotid artery. Occasionally, there is a bony bridge between the anterior and posterior clinoids. This can be recognized intraoperatively, and in this circumstance, total anterior clinoidectomy may be difficult or impossible.

After a full orbitozygomatic exposure is completed as described above, any remaining portion of the sphenoid wing is removed using rongeurs and burs. Using a high-speed drill and continuous irrigation, the optic canal is then carefully unroofed. Copious irrigation is necessary to prevent overheating of the optic nerve and resulting damage to vision. The entire length of the optic canal must be exposed for 180 degrees. Next, using exclusively diamond burs, the anterior clinoid is addressed. The central portion of the bone is removed, and drilling is extended along the lateral aspect of the optic canal. Drilling continues inferiorly until the main body of the clinoid is detached from the optic strut. At this point, the clinoid is free of all bony attachments. Small elevators are used to strip dura from the superior and lateral aspects of the clinoid. However, it is usually necessary to use a micro-cup forceps to actually remove the bone. Invariably, there is oozing of venous blood from the site of clinoid resection. This is controlled using Surgicel.

The dural opening is identical to that performed for the frontotemporal approach. Exposure of tumors along the medial sphenoid wing or at the tuberculum sella is augmented with careful attention to the sylvian fissure. Opening of the arachnoid along the anterior fissure, extending deep to reach the basal cisterns, aids in elevation of the frontal lobe. Wide opening of arachnoid spaces also promotes drainage of cerebrospinal fluid (CSF) and brain relaxation.

With removal of the anterior clinoid, the intradural space in the region of the basal cisterns is greatly enlarged. Despite the wide access to this area, however, the important anatomy may be obscured by tumor. Coagulation of the dural base is performed with great care and with attention to the likely location of the optic nerve at the optic canal and the carotid artery at the site of its exit from the cavernous sinus. Prior to addressing any tumor in the region of the optic canal, the dura of the canal is sharply opened using a nerve hook and scalpel. This step is critical to prevent deterioration of vision.

Further exposure of the proximal carotid artery, for example, for an aneurysm of the ophthalmic artery origin or carotid cave, necessitates mobilizing the carotid artery (i.e., dividing ring). After opening the dura, the distal ring can be cut or reflected from the artery; however, care must be taken to sharply incise the proximal ring (Pernezky's ring) as this is tightly adherent to the carotid artery adventitia and risks rupture if the surgeon attempts to reflect it from the artery per se. Usually, sharply cutting the ring laterally, leaving a cuff of the proximal ring adherent to the artery, allows for sufficient mobility.

The third cranial nerve can be readily followed from its cisternal section into the cavernous sinus, where its dural investment can be cut, using a similar technique as for cutting the falciform ligament and mobilizing the optic nerve as described above. This allows for the oculomotor nerve to be gently retracted and the medial contents of the cavernous sinus, including the carotid siphon and, lying just above the same, the abducens nerve, to be exposed. A temporary palsy is expected with even modest manipulation of CN III. The fourth cranial nerve lies lateral to CN III throughout the course of this exposure. It forms the medial border of Parkinson's triangle, the lateral border of which is V1.

The final step in the orbitozygomatic-transcavernous exposure is resection of the posterior clinoid process. Many of the same cautions and caveats provided with regard to drilling of the optic canal and anterior clinoid apply to the drilling of the posterior clinoid process as well. A 1-mm diamond drill is used under continuous irrigation during resection of the posterior clinoid. Its removal facilitates visualization of the basilar artery from the bifurcation to its midportion. In addition, the removal of the posterior clinoid provides exposure of the superior clivus and may be beneficial in approaching lesions such as a chordoma, though the extended middle fossa or Kawase approach, or an extended transsphenoidal approach may be preferable alternatives for tumors of the clivus.

◆ Postoperative Care and Complications

Patients should be counseled preoperatively to expect significant swelling of the ipsilateral eyelids; in the authors' experience this is more prominent when there is gross violation of the periorbita. This can usually be treated with simple conservative measures such as cold compresses. Enophthalmos is more likely to be encountered when excessive use of rongeurs is made in resecting the greater wing of the sphenoid and the roof of the orbit; removing as much as possible of these structures en bloc as described above allows for a good reconstruction of the orbit and minimizes this risk. Rarely, there may be entrapment of orbital contents by the replaced orbital flap; this may be particularly of concern if there is gross disruption of the periorbita. Patients should also be advised that they may experience pain with chewing; this is common and does not reflect disruption of the temporomandibular joint (TMJ), which should not be violated.

◆ Technical Pearls

- Elevate the scalp in the interfascial or subfascial plane to avoid injury to the frontal branch of the facial nerve.
- Dissect periorbita carefully using a sharp elevator to avoid herniation of orbital fat. Violation of the periorbita often cannot be entirely avoided.
- Pre-fit orbital rim microplates to facilitate proper anatomic alignment upon reconstruction.
- Do not blindly crack the orbital roof in cases of bony tumor involvement, because such cracking can be transmitted to the optic canal and can result in optic nerve injury.
- Tailor bony removal to the pathology. Many types of pathology in the anterior fossa do not require removal of the zygomatic arch.

◆ Conclusion

The orbitozygomatic approach and its principal variations discussed here greatly enhance visualization of intracranial structures that can be obtained through conventional frontotemporal or transsylvian approaches. The OZ approach can be readily tailored to suit the individual pathology, and can be effectively combined with other skull base approaches for exposure of the anterolateral skull base.

Suggested Readings

Hakuba A, Liu S, Nishimura S. The orbitozygomatic infratemporal approach: a new surgical technique. Surg Neurol 1986;26:271–276

Lemole GM Jr, Henn JS, Zabramski JM, Spetzler RF. Modifications to the orbitozygomatic approach. Technical note. J Neurosurg 2003;99:924–930

Schwartz MS, Anderson GJ, Horgan MA, Kellogg JX, McMenomey SO, Delashaw JB Jr. Quantification of increased exposure resulting from orbital rim and orbitozygomatic osteotomy via the frontotemporal transsylvian approach. J Neurosurg 1999;91:1020–1026

Seoane E, Tedeschi H, de Oliveira E, Wen HT, Rhoton AL Jr. The pretemporal transcavernous approach to the interpeduncular and prepontine cisterns: microsurgical anatomy and technique application. Neurosurgery 2000;46:891–898, discussion 898–899

Zabramski JM, Kiriş T, Sankhla SK, Cabiol J, Spetzler RF. Orbitozygomatic craniotomy. Technical note. J Neurosurg 1998;89:336–341

2

The Subtemporal Approach

Marc S. Schwartz

The subtemporal approach to skull base lesions may be utilized to gain access to pathology that extends along the floor of the middle fossa, including Meckel's cave. Trigeminal schwannomas with significant portions in Meckel's cave are the paradigmatic lesions for this approach. The elements of the subtemporal approach described in this section may also be combined with the petrosal approach to gain access to trigeminal schwannomas with both large Meckel's cave and posterior fossa components (dumbbell tumors) or petroclival meningiomas with significant extension along the floor of the middle fossa. Furthermore, the elements of the subtemporal approach can be combined with any of the infratemporal approaches to gain access to tumors that involve both the middle fossa and the infratemporal space, such as trigeminal neuromas extending along the third division through the foramen ovale and invasive skull base meningiomas.

◆ Surgical Anatomy

Superficially, the subtemporal approach requires mobilization of a large portion of the temporalis muscle to achieve access to the anterior reaches of the middle fossa. The temporalis originates from a large area of the temporal bone, runs beneath the arch of the zygoma, and inserts on the coronoid process of the mandible. The anterior aspect of the temporalis originates at the frontozygomatic process, which must be fully exposed. The temporal branch of the facial nerve overlies the temporalis fascia in this area, and injury to this branch can be avoided by maintaining dissection deep to the superficial layer of fascia.

The intracranial key to the performance of the subtemporal approach is an understanding of the anatomy of the petrous apex (Kawase's triangle). Bone removal is performed anterior to the internal auditory canal and cochlea, posterior to the mandibular branch of the trigeminal nerve, and medial to the carotid artery. The location of the carotid artery can be inferred from the greater superficial petrosal nerve, which overlies it on the floor of the middle fossa. An understanding of the anatomy of the trigeminal nerve itself is also critical, as this nerve can be traced to the foramina through which its second and third divisions pass (foramen rotundum and foramen ovale).

The subtemporal approach, as described, is considered an "extradural" approach. This is actually a misnomer, because Meckel's cave is an intradural space. The Meckel's cave dura, however, is an evagination of the posterior fossa dura. For that reason, this approach is extradural in relation to the middle fossa, whereas it is intradural in relation to the posterior fossa.

◆ Monitoring

Facial nerve and vestibulocochlear nerve monitoring is used for all cases, even if pathology does not extend into the posterior fossa, due to the possibility of encountering a dehiscent geniculate ganglion or superior semicircular canal during dural elevation. For large cases, especially with significant brainstem compression, somatosensory evoked potential monitoring may be used as well.

◆ Anesthetic Considerations

Serial compression devices are used for all patients. Cefuroxime, 1.5 g IV, is administered before the skin incision and repeated if the procedure lasts more than 8 hours. In addition to hyperventilation, intravenous mannitol is infused to facilitate brain relaxation. Muscle relaxation is not used to allow for facial nerve monitoring.

◆ Surgical Technique

The patient is placed in the supine position and is secured to the table so that it can be safely rotated. We utilize a Mayfield headholder and rigidly immobilize the patient's head rotated 45 to 60 degrees opposite the side of the lesion. Exposure and temporal lobe elevation may be facilitated by tilting the vertex slightly downward, although if there is extension of the lesion into the skull base and infratemporal space a more neutral position is maintained. The surgeon is seated at the head of the table. The scalp incision is similar to that made for the middle fossa approach; however, the anterior limb of the incision is carried forward to the hairline or beyond, in the case of a receding hairline (**Fig. 2.1**).

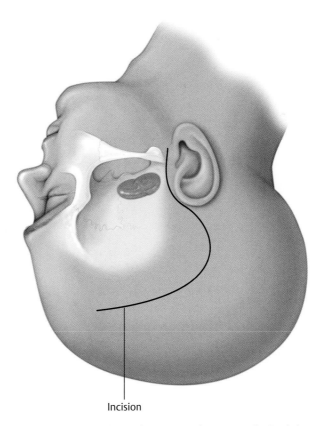

Incision

Fig. 2.1 Preauricular scalp incision. The anterior limb of the incision extends forward, at least to the hairline.

Extensive subgaleal elevation of the scalp is required to obtain adequate anterior exposure. Ideally, elevation is carried into the interfascial plane of the two-layer temporalis fascia. It is critical to maintain a plane deep to the fat pad that is consistently seen in this area to avoid injury of the temporal branch of the facial nerve. The root of the zygoma must also be exposed posteriorly. The temporalis fascia is incised just below the superior temporal line, and a relaxing incision is made through the fascia posteriorly. The temporalis muscle is elevated anteriorly. Subperiosteal dissection is performed to fully expose the zygoma at both its root and at the frontozygomatic process. Both the scalp and temporalis flaps can be held forward with perforating towel clips and rubber bands over a rolled sponge. Adequate retraction is necessary and can be facilitated by retracting to a Kerlix roll attached to the foot of the bed.

Although the craniotomy can be performed with bur holes and a craniotome, it is often safer to remove the bone flap entirely using cutting and diamond burs. Care is taken to achieve far-anterior and far-inferior removal of bone. The inferior extent of the craniotomy can be judged from the root of the zygoma, and anterosuperiorly the location of the sphenoid wing can be determined from the external shape of the skull. If the bone flap is performed too posterior or too superior, additional craniectomy can be performed after a cursory dural elevation. The temporalis muscle covers the entire area of bone removal and there is unlikely to be significant additional cosmetic problems (**Fig. 2.2**).

Extradural elevation is performed along the entire floor of the middle fossa extending anteriorly toward the temporal tip. Care is taken to identify the greater superficial petrosal nerve and the region of the geniculate ganglion, which may be dehiscent.

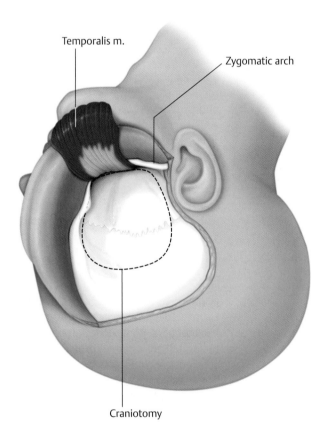

Temporalis m.

Zygomatic arch

Craniotomy

Fig. 2.2 Scalp and temporalis muscle flaps. The zygoma is exposed both at its root and at the frontozygomatic process. The bone flap is centered on the middle fossa and extends from the greater wing of the sphenoid to the floor of the middle fossa.

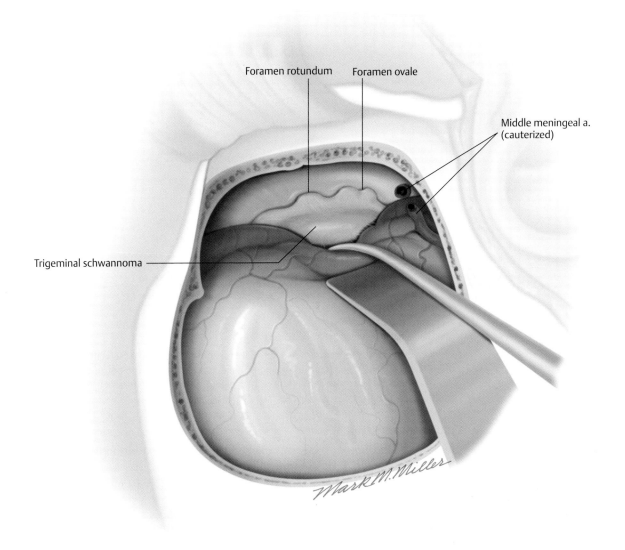

Fig. 2.3 Dural elevation along the floor of the middle fossa. Tumor can typically be palpated at the foramen ovale. The middle meningeal artery is sacrificed at the foramen spinosum.

Dissection in this area may be facilitated by exploring with a facial nerve stimulator using high stimulus intensity. Anterior exposure is augmented by coagulation and division of the middle meningeal artery at the foramen spinosum (**Fig. 2.3**). It may be necessary to pack this foramen to adequately control bleeding. We also use a diamond bur to fully expose the second and third divisions of the trigeminal nerve at their respective foramina. If possible, dural elevation is carried medially to the petrous apex in a manner identical to that done for the middle fossa approach. The bone in this area may be eroded by a schwannoma or other expansile tumor, and care must be taken to recognize and avoid injury to the carotid artery if it is dehiscent. The temporal lobe is elevated extradurally using a self-retaining retractor.

The bone of the petrous apex, lateral to the greater superficial petrosal nerve, eustachian tube, and carotid artery, is carefully removed using diamond burs and continuous irrigation. In cases of trigeminal schwannoma, much of this bone may be eroded tumor, and not much drilling is necessary. However, it is necessary to completely

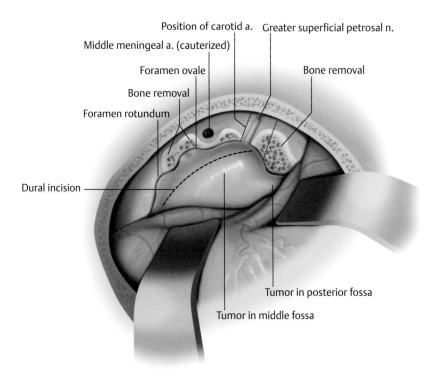

Fig. 2.4   The dura propria of Meckel's cave is exposed. This step is facilitated by the presence of a large schwannoma. Drilling of bone is performed at the petrous apex to gain access to the posterior fossa. If the tumor extends through the foramen ovale or spinosum, bone is drilled to gain access to these locations.

remove this portion of bone, especially if there is any extension of tumor into the posterior fossa (**Fig. 2.4**). With meningiomas, this drilling may be more difficult, but drilling is made even more important as it will serve to partially devascularize the tumor.

For trigeminal schwannomas located primarily in Meckel's cave, access to the tumor is attained by direct dissection via the dura propria (dura of Meckel's cave, derived from the posterior fossa) at the foramen ovale. As the temporal lobe dura is gently elevated, sharp technique is used to come through the thin tissue overlying the nerve. Tumor can be directly debulked (**Fig. 2.5**).

An attempt is made to preserve as many trigeminal fibers as possible. When the main trunk of the trigeminal nerve is located medial to tumor bulk, most fibers can be preserved. When tumor is medial, however, preservation of fibers is more difficult. After removal of the main bulk of tumor from Meckel's cave, the trigeminal nerve can be followed peripherally into extradural spaces or centrally into the posterior fossa. Usually, corridors of access are widened, facilitating a limited exposure in any direction. For extension of tumor into the posterior fossa, access is improved by a more anterior to posterior trajectory (**Fig. 2.6**). Of course, if there is a large mass of tumor in the posterior fossa, the subtemporal approach can be combined with a petrosal approach to safely resect tumor in its entirety.

For meningiomas, tumor may extend intradurally in both the middle and posterior fossae. For these cases, the approach is individualized, including the combination of the subtemporal approach with either an extended middle fossa or a combined petrosal approach. We would generally recommend dural opening into the posterior fossa first, to drain cerebrospinal fluid (CSF) and relax the brain. Opening in this area can be accomplished in a fashion similar to that used for middle fossa craniotomy.

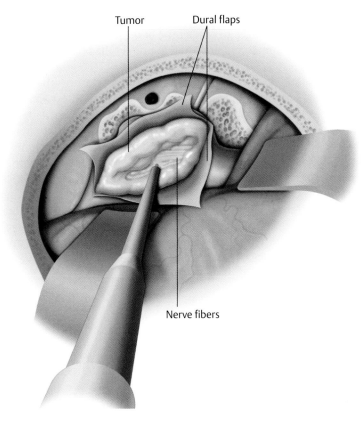

Tumor   Dural flaps

Nerve fibers

Fig. 2.5   The dura propria of Meckel's cave is opened, providing direct access to the tumor and to trigeminal nerve fibers.

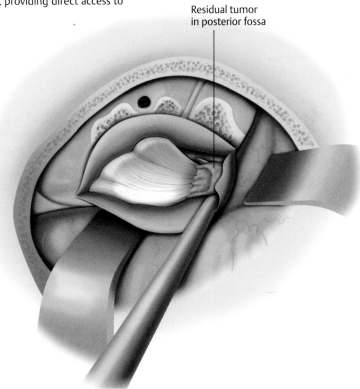

Residual tumor in posterior fossa

Fig. 2.6   After debulking of the tumor, the dural opening is extended into the posterior fossa. The tumor can be delivered from the posterior fossa via this dural opening and the widened entrance to Meckel's cave.

Dural opening into the middle fossa is performed just lateral to the edge of tumor. We prefer to leave the lateral dura in place to protect the brain. Cottonoids are advanced to develop the plane between tumor and brain and to protect the brain during tumor resection.

After resection of tumor and the establishment of hemostasis, closure is performed. Generally, we would not advocate primary dural closure. An onlay collagenous material may be used to reconstruct the middle fossa dura if it has been opened. When intradural exposure has been performed and there is communication with mastoid air cells or the middle ear, abdominal fat is used to fill the drilled portion of temporal bone. For extradural cases or those in which there is no communication with the aerodigestive system, the use of fat is unnecessary. The bone plate is held in anatomic position using titanium microplates, and the temporalis fascia is sutured. In most cases, it is advisable to pull the body of the temporalis muscle anteriorly and to make certain there is adequate muscle bulk in the frontozygomatic region to minimize the cosmetic issues associated with temporal wasting. The scalp may be closed over a subgaleal drain, which is left in place for several days, to prevent postoperative periorbital swelling.

◆ Technical Pearls

- Dissection is facilitated by the presence of a large tumor bulk in Meckel's cave.
- Fully debulk tumor in Meckel's cave before approaching the posterior fossa or infratemporal portion.
- Drain CSF via Meckel's cave before entering the posterior fossa.
- Active temporal retraction is often not necessary after CSF is drained.
- Meningiomas and other skull base lesions may be more challenging than trigeminal schwannomas.

◆ Conclusion

The subtemporal approach provides excellent access to the Meckel's cave region. Morbidity is minimized, as this is primarily an extradural approach. Dissection is actually facilitated by the presence of a trigeminal schwannoma, and the approach and subsequent tumor resection may be easier for a larger tumor than for a smaller tumor. Although this approach can also be considered for other lesions, such as skull base meningiomas, it is perhaps best suited for trigeminal nerve tumors with the major part in Meckel's cave.

Suggested Readings

Hsu FP, Anderson GJ, Dogan A, et al. Extended middle fossa approach: quantitative analysis of petroclival exposure and surgical freedom as a function of successive temporal bone removal by using frameless stereotaxy. J Neurosurg 2004;100(4):695–699

Kawase T, Shiobara R, Toya S. Anterior transpetrosal-transtentorial approach for sphenopetroclival meningiomas: surgical method and results in 10 patients. Neurosurgery 1991;28(6):869–875, discussion 875–876

Yoshida K, Kawase T. Trigeminal neurinomas extending into multiple fossae: surgical methods and review of the literature. J Neurosurg 1999;91(2):202–211

Youssef S, Kim EY, Aziz KM, Hemida S, Keller JT, van Loveren HR. The subtemporal interdural approach to dumbbell-shaped trigeminal schwannomas: cadaveric prosection. Neurosurgery 2006; 59(4, Suppl 2)ONS270–ONS277, discussion ONS277–ONS278

3

The Middle Cranial Fossa Approach to Vestibular Schwannomas

Rick A. Friedman and Jose N. Fayad

For decades, gaining access to the cerebellopontine angle and the prepontine cisterns has presented a formidable challenge. Several conventional neurosurgical approaches to this region have been described, including the subtemporal and transsylvian, and a combined approach incorporating both techniques. Modern skull base approaches, including the middle cranial fossa approach and the middle fossa transpetrous approach, have been instrumental in removing the petrous barrier. This chapter describes the utility of the middle cranial fossa approach for removing vestibular schwannomas of less than 2 cm in patients with useful hearing.

◆ Overview

Approaches designed to expose vestibular schwannomas, petroclival meningiomas, chondromas, chondrosarcomas, and chordomas involving the petrous apex and clivus must take into consideration the vital neighboring neurovascular structures. The risks encountered in the region of the prepontine cistern during the management of aneurysms of the posterior circulation were best described by Drake in 1961: "The upper clival region is to be considered no-man's land." Several conventional neurosurgical approaches to this region have been described, including the subtemporal and transsylvian and a combination half-and-half approach incorporating both techniques. Despite advances in microsurgical techniques and neuroanesthesia, the petrous bone has previously been an impediment to satisfactory exposure in this anatomically complex region. Modern skull base approaches, including the middle fossa and the middle fossa transpetrous, have been instrumental in removing the petrous apex barrier, minimizing temporal lobe retraction, and improving the line of sight to this region.

The middle fossa approach was first described in the literature in 1904. The sentinel work of William F. House in 1961 led to the refinement of this approach to the internal auditory canal (IAC) and the cerebellopontine angle (CPA). The approach was used initially for the decompression of the IAC in cases of extensive otosclerosis involving the labyrinthine bone. That indication was abandoned, but the middle fossa approach has become a workhorse in our approach to small vestibular schwannomas, petroclival meningiomas, and chordoma/chondrosarcoma (**Table 3.1**).

◆ Surgical Anatomy

The surgical anatomy of the temporal bone from the middle fossa approach is complex (**Figs. 3.1 and 3.2**). Landmarks are not as apparent as with other approaches

Table 3.1   Indications for the Middle Fossa Approach
Vestibular schwannoma (<2 cm)
Petroclival meningioma
Chondroma
Chondrosarcoma
Chondroblastoma
Chordoma
Trigeminal schwannoma
Infraclinoidal basilar tip aneurysms

through the temporal bone. Laboratory dissection is essential so that the surgeon may become familiar with the anatomy from above.

Anteriorly, the limit of the dissection is the middle meningeal artery, which is anterior and lateral to the greater superficial petrosal nerve. Excessive anterior retraction can lead to postoperative paresthesias in V3. The arcuate eminence roughly marks the position of the superior semicircular canal. The relationship between the

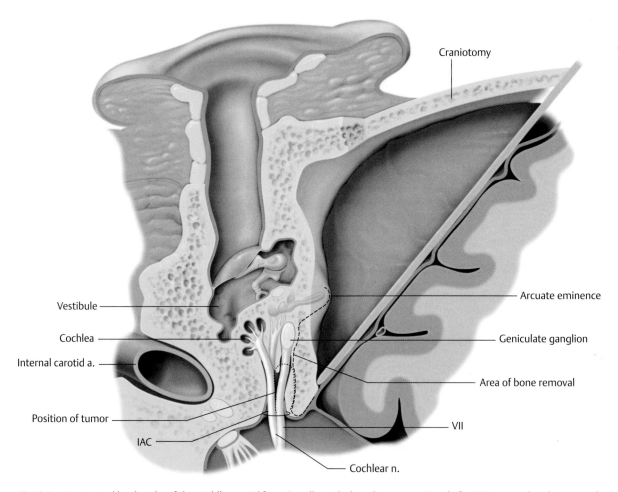

Fig. 3.1 Anatomical landmarks of the middle cranial fossa (small vestibular schwannoma in relief). EAC, external auditory canal; IAC, internal auditory canal.

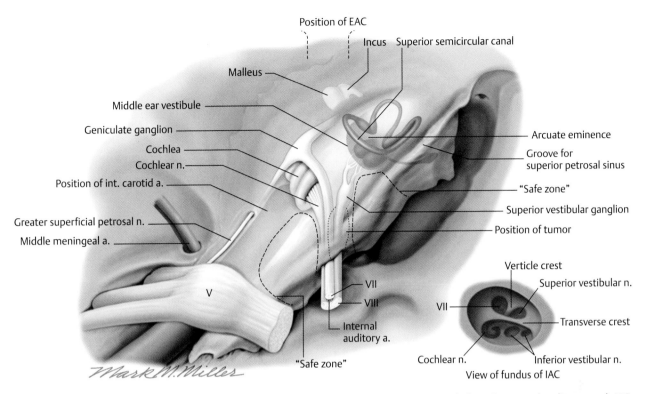

Fig. 3.2 Anatomical landmarks of the middle cranial fossa (small vestibular schwannoma in relief). EAC, external auditory canal; IAC, internal auditory canal.

arcuate eminence and the superior semicircular canal is inconstant. The superior semicircular canal tends to be perpendicular to the petrous ridge. Medially, the superior petrosal sinus runs along the petrous ridge.

Surgical tolerances are tight in the area of the lateral IAC. The labyrinthine portion of the facial nerve lies immediately posterior to the basal turn of the cochlea. Bill's bar separates the facial and superior vestibular nerves. Slightly posterior and lateral to this area is the vestibule and ampullated end of the superior semicircular canal.

Identification of the geniculate ganglion can be accomplished by tracing the greater superficial petrosal nerve posteriorly. The ganglion is dehiscent in approximately 16% of patients.

The IAC lies roughly on the same axis as the external auditory canal; this relationship is useful in orienting the surgical field. The area around the porus acusticus medially is a "safe zone" in comparison to the lateral or fundal region and provides an excellent place to begin IAC dissection. We begin our dissection medially, by drilling in the meatal plane in the area of the bisection of the angle formed by the superior semicircular canal and the greater superficial petrosal nerve. The IAC can be located initially in this medial area of the temporal bone and followed laterally.

◆ Surgical Technique

Administer preoperative antibiotics and continue them for 24 hours postoperatively. Intraoperative furosemide and mannitol are given to allow easier temporal lobe retraction. The authors administer dexamethasone intravenously during the procedure and continue this for 24 hours postoperatively. Long-acting muscle relaxants are avoided during surgery so as not to interfere with facial nerve monitoring.

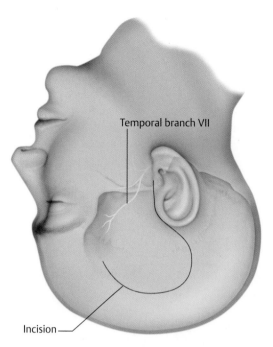

Fig. 3.3 Preauricular/temporal scalp incision. Note position of the frontal branch of cranial nerve VII.

The patient is placed in the supine position with the head turned to the side opposite the lesion. The surgeon is seated at the head of the table and the anesthesiologist at the foot. An incision is made in the preauricular area and extended superiorly in a gently curving fashion. *Care must be taken near the anterior extension of the incision to avoid injury to the frontal branch of the facial nerve* (**Fig. 3.3**). The temporalis muscle is incised, beginning at the zygomatic root, along the linea temporalis, and the muscle is elevated from the temporal fossa and reflected anteroinferiorly. This exposes the temporal squama.

Utilizing cutting and diamond burs, a temporal craniotomy is performed. The craniotomy measures approximately 5 × 5 cm and is two-thirds anterior and one-third posterior to the zygomatic root (**Fig. 3.4**). The inferior limit of the flap should be at the level of the zygoma, approximating the floor of the middle cranial fossa. Care must be taken to avoid laceration of the underlying dura. The bone flap is set aside for later replacement.

The dura is elevated from the floor of the middle fossa. The initial landmark is the middle meningeal artery, which marks the anterior extent of the dissection. Frequently, venous bleeding is encountered from this area and can be controlled with oxidized cellulose (Surgicel). Elevation of the dura proceeds in a posterior-to-anterior fashion. As stated above, in approximately 16% of cases the geniculate ganglion of the facial nerve is dehiscent, and injury can be avoided with posterior-to-anterior dural elevation. The petrous ridge is identified, and care is taken not to lacerate the superior petrosal sinus, as it is elevated from its sulcus. The arcuate eminence and greater superficial petrosal nerve are identified and the House-Urban retractor is placed (**Fig. 3.5**). These are the major landmarks for the subsequent intratemporal dissection.

When the dura has been elevated, typically with a suction irrigator and a blunt dural elevator, the House-Urban retractor is placed to support the temporal lobe. *To maintain a secure position, the teeth of the retaining retractor should be locked against the bone margins of the craniotomy window and the retractor blade must be placed on the true petrous ridge.* Using a large diamond bur and continuous suction irrigation, the

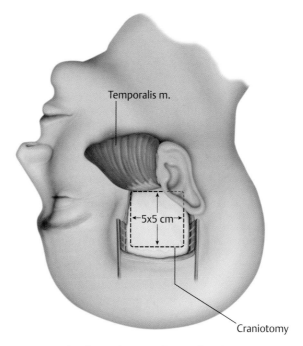

Fig. 3.4 Skin flap and temporalis muscle reflected demonstrating the outline of the temporal craniotomy.

superior semicircular canal is identified, but not blue-lined, at the arcuate eminence. The superior semicircular canal makes a 45- to 60-degree angle with the IAC (**Fig. 3.6**).

Bone removal over the IAC begins medially at the porus acusticus with a large diamond bur. The area of bone anteromedial to the IAC and medial to the petrous carotid

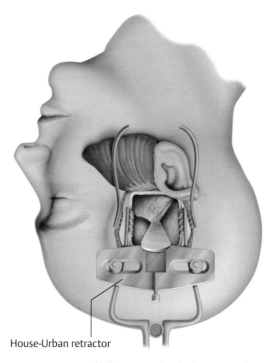

Fig. 3.5 Temporal lobe retracted with the House-Urban retractor placed in the true petrous ridge after elevation of the superior petrosal sinus within the dura.

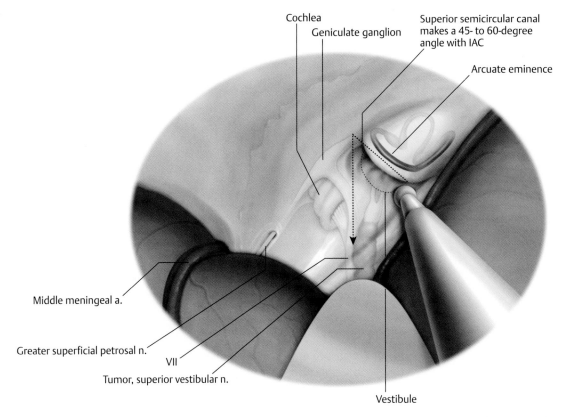

Cochlea

Geniculate ganglion

Superior semicircular canal
makes a 45- to 60-degree
angle with IAC

Arcuate eminence

Middle meningeal a.

Greater superficial petrosal n.

VII

Tumor, superior vestibular n.

Vestibule

Fig. 3.6   Critical microanatomical landmarks. Diamond ball no greater than 2.0 mm can be safely used to remove the bone of the lateral IAC.

artery can be saucerized, exposing its anterior surface. Next the bone in the "post-meatal triangle" can be removed exposing the posterior surface of the IAC. Medially, 270 degrees of bone can be removed from its circumference (**Fig. 3.7**). The circumference of the IAC is less exposed laterally because of the location of the inner ear. The lateral end of the IAC is dissected with clear identification of the labyrinthine segment of the facial nerve, Bill's bar, and the superior vestibular nerve.

The labyrinthine portion of the facial nerve is identified proximal to the ganglion. Care must be taken to avoid the cochlea, which lies ≤1 mm anterior to the labyrinthine portion of the facial nerve. This is best accomplished by careful delineation of the anterior limit of the IAC with a blunt hook. *The superior vestibular nerve can be followed laterally approximately one-half the distance of the labyrinthine facial nerve to avoid entering the ampulla of the superior semicircular canal* (**Fig. 3.7**). The lateral dissection is essential for clear identification of the facial nerve and complete removal of tumor from the fundus of the IAC.

The dura of the IAC is divided along the posterior portion of the IAC (**Fig. 3.8**). The facial nerve is identified in the anterior portion of the IAC (**Fig. 3.9**). Tumor dissection begins in a medial-to-lateral direction to avoid avulsion of the cochlear nerve fibers at the habenula perforata. The superior vestibular nerve is sectioned, and the tumor is separated from the facial and cochlear nerves. Using a right-angled hook, the inferior vestibular nerve is divided, and the tumor is delivered gently from the cochlear and facial nerves and removed (**Figs. 3.10 and 3.11**). To preserve hearing, the internal auditory artery must be preserved. The vessel typically runs between the facial and the cochlear nerves but is not visible during the dissection. Keys to successful exposure and outcomes are listed below (see Technical Pearls).

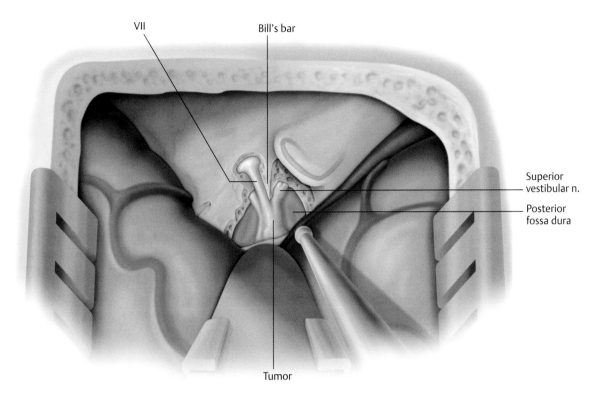

Fig. 3.7 Essential bone removal at the lateral IAC. The facial nerve is followed to the geniculate ganglion and the superior vestibular nerve is exposed for one-half the distance of the labyrinthine facial nerve. Bill's bar is clearly defined. The distance from the cochlear base to the ampulla of the superior semicircular canal is roughly 2.5 mm. This limits the size of bur used during dissection at the lateralmost area.

After irrigation of the tumor bed and establishment of hemostasis, abdominal fat is used to close the defect in the IAC. The wound is closed with absorbable subcutaneous sutures over a Penrose drain. This drain typically is removed on the first postoperative day. A mastoid-type pressure dressing is maintained for 3 days postoperatively.

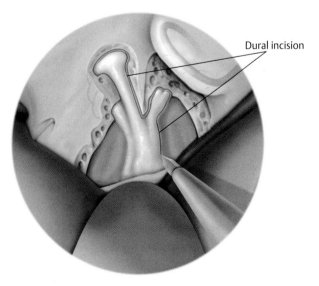

Fig. 3.8 The posterior dural incision over the tumor is reflected anteriorly.

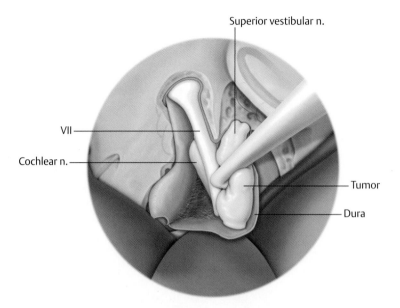

Fig. 3.9   The facial nerve is fully delineated and dissected free from the tumor prior to tumor removal.

The patient is observed in the intensive care unit for the first postoperative day and typically is hospitalized for 4 to 5 days. When the patient leaves the intensive care unit, ambulation is encouraged. We believe that early ambulation is important for rapid vestibular compensation.

Variation: The Extended Middle Cranial Fossa Approach

The middle fossa approach can be extended to gain wider access to the prepontine cistern and premeatal posterior cranial fossa. This is often necessary when lesions of the temporal bone extend to the clivus, for larger schwannomas involving the fifth or eighth nerve, petroclival meningiomas, and aneurysms of the infraclinoidal basilar

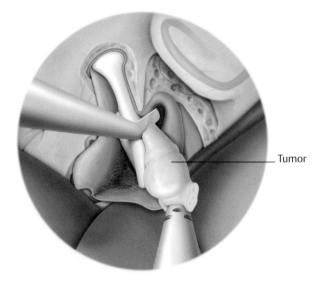

Fig. 3.10   The tumor is being removed after freeing it medially. It is dissected from medial to lateral with extreme care in the region of the fundus beneath the transverse crest.

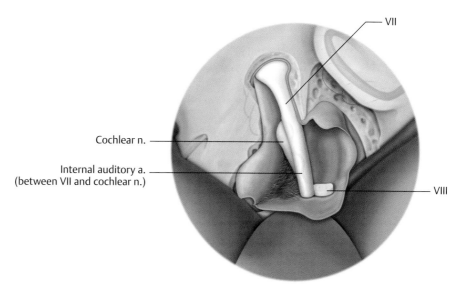

Fig. 3.11 The internal canal contents after tumor removal, demonstrating the remaining contents. This defect is subsequently packed with abdominal fat.

tip. The area of bone removed comprises the entire petrous apex from the IAC posteriorly to the internal carotid artery (ICA) laterally and the petroclival junction anteromedially. Inferiorly the bone removal extends to the inferior petrosal sinus limiting access to lesions of the lower one third of the clivus (**Fig. 3.12**).

The middle fossa floor is exposed extradurally with identification of the middle meningeal artery at the foramen spinosum, the greater superficial petrosal nerve at the facial hiatus and along the petrosal ridge, the arcuate eminence, and the mandibular

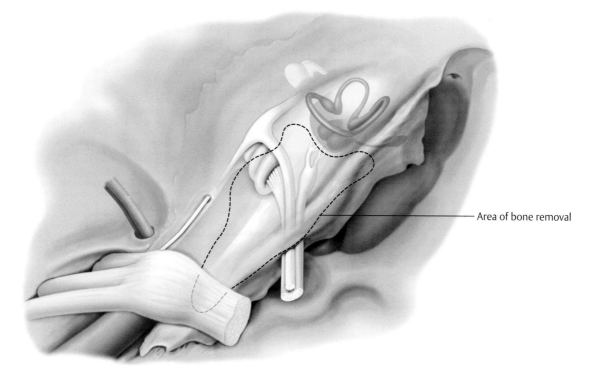

Fig. 3.12 Area of bone removal for the extended middle cranial fossa approach.

branch of the trigeminal nerve (**Fig. 3.12**). The middle meningeal artery is sacrificed, and the horizontal segment of the petrous ICA is exposed. After placement of the temporal lobe retractor, bone removal is initiated medially in the area of the porus acusticus, at an approximately 60 degree angle to the arcuate eminence or on a line bisecting the angle subtended by the arcuate eminence and the greater superficial petrosal nerve. The IAC is skeletonized in its entirety with preservation of the cochlea and the superior semicircular canal. The exposure gained is limited by the petrous carotid artery anterolaterally and the posterior fossa dura posteromedially. The inferior limit of the dissection is the inferior petrosal sinus in the petro-occipital suture.

The dura is opened along the inferior edge of the temporal lobe. The subtemporal dura is sectioned perpendicular to the dural opening directly to the segment of the superior petrosal sinus exposed by the bone removed from the anterior petrous dissection. The superior petrosal sinus is sectioned between two titanium clips, exposing the junction of the posterior fossa dura and the tentorium cerebelli (**Figs. 3.13 and 3.14**). The posterior fossa dura is opened to the apex of the anterior petrosectomy. The tentorium cerebelli is sectioned to a point posterior to the entry of the trochlear nerve, to the tentorial edge. Care must be taken during this step to avoid sectioning the tentorium too far posteriorly and inadvertently injuring the vein of Labbé as it enters the transverse sinus. The combination of the extended middle cranial fossa and the translabyrinthine approaches provides wide exposure of the CPA and prepontine region without the need for facial nerve rerouting.

Fig. 3.13   (A,B) Dural incisions. ICA, internal carotid artery.

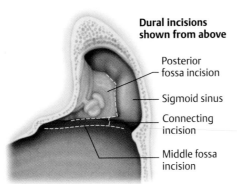

Dural incisions shown from above

Posterior fossa incision

Sigmoid sinus

Connecting incision

Middle fossa incision

A

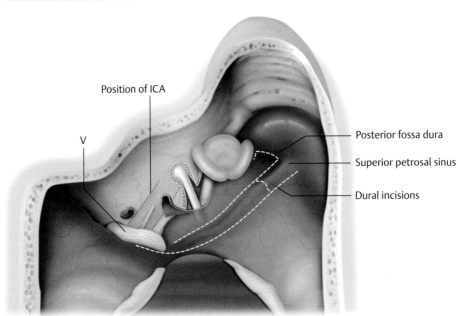

Position of ICA

V

Posterior fossa dura

Superior petrosal sinus

Dural incisions

B

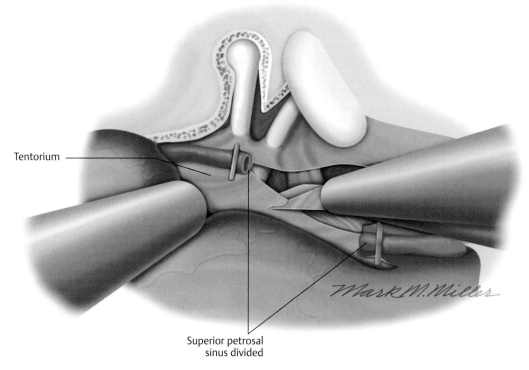

Tentorium

Superior petrosal
sinus divided

Fig. 3.14 The superior petrosal sinus is clipped and divided. The lateral-to-medial incision of the tentorium extends to the notch. Care must be taken to incise posteriorly within the notch to protect the trochlear nerve as it enters the tentorium anteriorly. Additionally, the surgeon must consider the vein of Labbé, as in some instances it travels with the leaves of the tentorium.

◆ Limitations

The limitations of the middle fossa approach are dictated by the tumor type and the regional anatomy. The middle cranial fossa approach has virtually eliminated the barrier imposed by the petrous apex when approaching lesions of the posterior cranial fossa within and anterior to the IAC. This approach is an essential part of tumor removal with hearing and facial nerve functional preservation. Although hearing preservation is possible with all of the tumors listed in **Table 3.1**, hearing preservation is extremely unlikely with vestibular schwannomas larger than 2 cm (**Table 3.2**).

Anatomically, the middle cranial fossa approach provides superb access to lesions of the IAC and prepontine cistern down to the level of the inferior petrosal sinus. Lesions posterior to the IAC are difficult to access through this approach alone and often

Table 3.2 Factors Affecting Hearing Preservation in Vestibular Schwannoma
Limited intracanalicular extension
Tumor size (<2 cm)
ABR IT5 <0.4 milliseconds
Video/nystagmagram (VNG) suggesting a tumor arising from the superior vestibular nerve
Word recognition >70%
Cerebrospinal fluid in the fundus on T2-weighted magnetic resonance imaging confirming a more medially placed tumor

require a combined petrosal approach. Combining posterior access via a retrolaby-rinthine or translabyrinthine approach with an extended middle fossa approach provides outstanding access to most areas of the posterior fossa, except the lower clivus, without the need for facial nerve rerouting.

◆ Technical Pearls

- Avoid the frontal branch of the facial nerve (**Fig. 3.1**).
- Place the retractor blade in the true petrous ridge.
- Define the anterior limit of the IAC from the porus to the fundus.
- Completely delineate the vertical crest.
- Sharply dissect the tumor from medial to lateral.

◆ Conclusion

The middle cranial fossa approach is an invaluable approach to tumors of the IAC and lesions of the petrous apex and prepontine cistern. This approach affords access to complex tumors while potentially preserving hearing. The middle cranial fossa approach to vestibular schwannoma removal is our approach of choice for patients with small tumors (≤2 cm) and serviceable hearing. We have shown the safety and efficacy of this approach for hearing preservation surgery.

Suggested Readings
Drake CG. Bleeding aneurysms of the basilar artery. Direct surgical management in four cases. J Neuro-surg 1961;18:230–238
House WF. Surgical exposure of the internal auditory canal and its contents through the middle, cra-nial fossa. Laryngoscope 1961;71:1363–1385
House WF, Hitselberger WE, Horn KL. The middle fossa transpetrous approach to the anterior-superior cerebellopontine angle. Am J Otol 1986;7:1–4

4

The Infracochlear/ Infralabyrinthine Approach to the Petrous Apex

Derald E. Brackmann and J. Walter Kutz, Jr.

Before the antibiotic era, infections were the most common lesions of the petrous apex and they carried a high mortality rate. Fortunately, with the advent of antibiotics, infections of the petrous apex are rarely observed by the neurotologist. Instead, most lesions of the petrous apex are cystic in nature and can be successfully treated with the same drainage procedures previously developed for infections. With the advent of high-resolution computed tomography (CT), the precise location of the lesion and an appropriate approach can be planned. This chapter describes the infralabyrinthine and infracochlear approaches to cystic lesions of the petrous apex.

◆ Evaluation

Lesions of the petrous apex present with a wide range of symptoms. The classic presentation of infection of the petrous apex is Gradenigo's syndrome, which is characterized by the triad of otorrhea, retro-orbital pain, and an ipsilateral abducens nerve palsy. In noninfectious lesions, hearing loss and dizziness are more common presentations. Cystic lesions may occasionally cause facial spasm or paresis, but facial nerve paralysis is more consistent with a neoplastic process. Pain in the form of otalgia, retro-orbital pain, and headaches is a common finding and is dependent on the location of the lesion.

Recent advancements in imaging have had a significant impact on the diagnosis and treatment of petrous apex lesions. High-resolution CT gives superb bony detail of the lesion and the surrounding vital structures that dictate the appropriate approach to these lesions. Magnetic resonance imaging (MRI) enhanced with gadolinium contrast gives excellent soft tissue detail and can diagnose most lesions without the need for tissue. **Table 4.1** lists the typical appearance of petrous apex lesions on CT and MRI.

Approaches to the petrous apex are based on the various air cell tracts of the temporal bone. Air cell tracts superior to the otic capsule can be approached through the middle fossa, superior semicircular canal, the attic, or the zygomatic root. Anterior approaches are based on the air cell tracts between the cochlea, middle fossa dura, and carotid artery. However, the most common contemporary approaches are based on the air cell tracts inferior to the labyrinth and include the infralabyrinthine and infracochlear approaches.

◆ Preoperative Workup

Appropriate imaging should be obtained and generally includes both CT and MRI to fully characterize the lesion and surgical approach. A full audiometric evaluation is

Table 4.1 Imaging Characteristics of Lesions of the Petrous Apex

Lesion	CT	MRI T1-Weighted	MRI T2-Weighted	Gadolinium-Enhanced
Petrous apex marrow asymmetry	Normal bony architecture	Hyperintense	Hypointense	No
Retained mucus	Normal bony architecture	Hypointense	Hyperintense	No
Mucocele	Smooth erosion	Hypointense	Hyperintense	No
Cholesterol granuloma	Smooth erosion	Hyperintense	Hyperintense	No
Epidermoid cyst	Loss of air cells, expansile	Hypointense	Hyperintense	No
Chordoma/chondrosarcoma	Bone destruction, occasional calcifications	Hypointense to isointense	Hyperintense	Yes
Metastatic lesion	Bone destruction	Hypointense to isointense	Hyperintense	Yes
Internal carotid artery aneurism	Erosion of carotid canal, calcifications	Hypointense	Mixed	Rim

obtained including air, bone, and speech reception thresholds because it is essential to document preoperative hearing in any procedure that may jeopardize hearing. A videonystagmogram (VNG) is obtained in patients who present with vertigo or imbalance. Patients are counseled regarding the expectations from surgery. It is emphasized that the procedure is a drainage procedure and may not entirely relieve symptoms and may require additional procedures. Preoperative cranial nerve deficits usually improve after drainage of cystic lesions; however, long-standing deficits are less likely to respond to surgery.

The choice of approach depends on multiple factors. In patients without serviceable hearing, a translabyrinthine approach provides the safest and most direct access to the petrous apex. In patients with hearing, the infralabyrinthine, infracochlear, or transsphenoidal approaches are appropriate. A high jugular bulb is an obstacle for drainage of petrous apex cysts using the infralabyrinthine approach. The infracochlear approach places the carotid artery at risk and should be attempted by a surgeon with intimate knowledge of the anatomy of the hypotympanum. The infracochlear approach has the advantage of avoiding a mastoidectomy and places the drainage site closer to the eustachian tube. The transsphenoidal approach places the carotid artery and optic nerve at risk; however, the use of intraoperative image guidance has made this approach safer.

◆ Infralabyrinthine Approach to the Petrous Apex

Surgical Anatomy

The boundaries of the infralabyrinthine approach are the posterior semicircular canal superiorly, the jugular bulb and sigmoid sinus inferiorly and posteriorly, and the facial nerve anteriorly. Preoperative imaging should be utilized to determine the position of the jugular bulb because a high jugular bulb may restrict access to the petrous apex through this approach and another approach should be considered.

Surgical Technique

The patient is placed supine with the head turned away from the operative side. Intraoperative facial nerve monitoring is utilized. A standard postauricular incision is made 1 cm posterior to the postauricular sulcus. A second incision is made through the periosteum from the zygomatic root along the linea temporalis and then carried inferior to the mastoid tip. The periosteum is elevated until the posterior extent of the external auditory canal is identified. A simple mastoidectomy is performed and the middle fossa plate, sigmoid sinus, and facial nerve are identified. The sigmoid sinus is followed until the jugular bulb is identified. The superior aspect of the jugular bulb is the inferior limit of this approach. Next the posterior semicircular canal and the posterior half of the lateral semicircular canal are skeletonized, taking care not to expose the membranous labyrinth. Once the jugular bulb and posterior semicircular canal have been identified, the air cell tracts are followed using diamond burs and curettes until the cystic lesion is entered (**Fig. 4.1**).

The opening is widened using the anatomic limits, and all loose debris is removed from the cyst using suction and irrigation. The largest silicone tubing possible is placed in the surgical tract to prevent stenosis (**Fig. 4.2**). The periosteum is reapproximated using absorbable sutures, and the skin is closed in the standard fashion. A pressure dressing is placed and left in place for 24 hours.

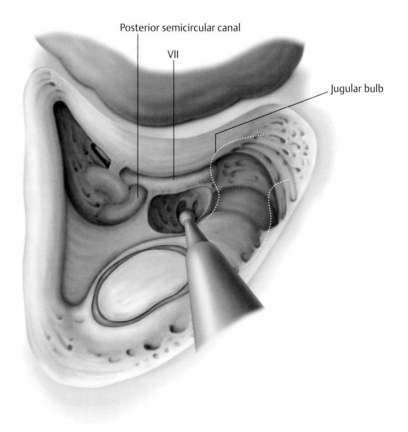

Fig. 4.1 The posterior lateral semicircular canal, posterior semicircular canal, and jugular bulb have been identified and are the boundaries of the approach.

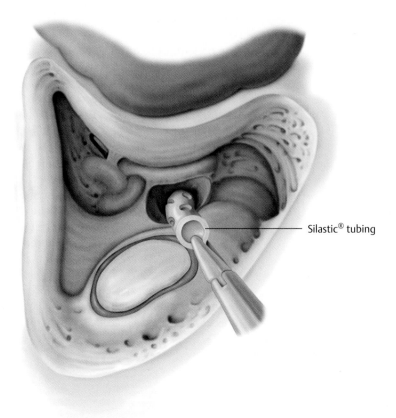

Silastic® tubing

Fig. 4.2   The petrous apex has been entered, the opening enlarged, and a piece of Silastic tubing placed.

Pitfalls

The infralabyrinthine approach offers direct access to the petrous apex; however, injury to vital structures may result in complications that should be managed appropriately. A small tear in the jugular bulb can usually be managed with oxidized cellulose or Gelfoam soaked with thrombin. However, more significant injuries to the bulb may require packing of the bulb. Large sheets of oxidized cellulose are used to pack the lumen of the jugular bulb through the tear. Small pieces of packing should not be placed near the opening to prevent possible embolization. Fistulas of the lateral and posterior semicircular canals should be recognized promptly. Careful inspection should be performed without suctioning directly over the defect. A small piece of fascia can be placed over the defect and secured with bone wax. A small defect detected early may not result in hearing loss; however, patients may complain of postoperative vertigo. Stenosis of the surgical tract may occur and can be best avoided by creating as large an opening as possible and by placement of a Silastic tube to stent the tract.

◆ Transcanal Infracochlear Approach to the Petrous Apex

Surgical Anatomy

The boundaries of the infracochlear approach include the cochlea, the jugular bulb, the facial nerve, and the petrous carotid artery. Identification of these structures is essential to safely perform this approach. The bone of the inferior and anterior bony tympanic annulus must be sufficiently removed to gain adequate access to the hypotympanum. Injuries to the cochlea are prevented by staying inferior to the round window. The facial nerve can be identified by following the chorda tympani nerve inferiorly and posteriorly. The carotid artery and jugular bulb should be identified before more medial dissection continues.

Surgical Technique

The patient is placed supine with the head turned away from the operative side. Facial nerve monitoring is utilized. A standard postauricular incision is made 1 cm posterior to the postauricular sulcus. A second incision is made through the periosteum from the zygomatic root along the linea temporalis and then carried inferior to the mastoid tip. The external auditory canal is transected at the bony-cartilaginous junction (**Fig. 4.3**). A tympanomeatal flap is then elevated from the 2 o'clock and the 10 o'clock positions. The tympanomeatal flap is left attached at the umbo and superior canal wall. The hypotympanum is furthered exposed by removing the bony external auditory canal anteriorly and inferiorly (**Fig. 4.4**). The chorda tympani nerve is followed posteriorly and inferiorly to find the facial nerve and the posterior limit of the approach (**Fig. 4.5**). The bone of the hypotympanum is carefully removed until the carotid artery and jugular bulb are clearly delineated (**Fig. 4.6**). The superior limit of the approach is a line perpendicular to the round window to prevent inadvertent injury to the cochlea. Jacobsen's nerve can be followed inferiorly to the bone separating the jugular bulb and carotid artery. The removal of air cells now continues medial until the cyst is entered. The opening should be widened as much as possible using the carotid artery, jugular bulb, and basal turn of the cochlea as the limits. A piece of Silastic tubing is then placed to prevent stenosis of the surgical tract (**Fig. 4.7**). Bone pate is used to repair the defect in the bony canal wall, and the soft tissue of the external auditory canal is returned to its normal position (**Fig. 4.8**). The external auditory canal is packed with gelatin sponge and the postauricular incision is closed.

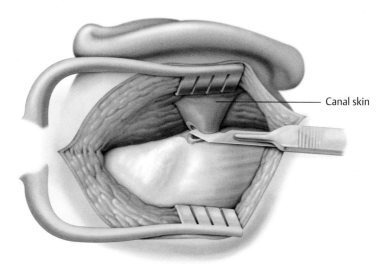

Canal skin

Fig. 4.3 Depiction of the infralabyrinthine approach to the petrous apex. Note how a high jugular bulb prevents access to the petrous apex using this approach.

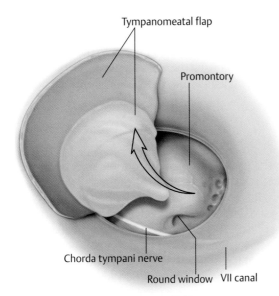

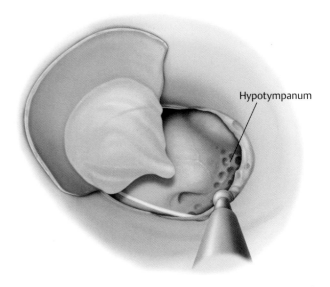

Fig. 4.4 The tympanomeatal flap is left attached to the superior bony canal and umbo, allowing a view into the hypotympanum.

Fig. 4.5 A tympanomeatal flap is elevated with incision at the 2 and 10 o'clock positions.

Pitfalls

Familiarity with the anatomy of the hypotympanum is essential to prevent injury to vital structures in a relatively confined space. Treatments of injuries to the jugular bulb are detailed in the previous section on the infralabyrinthine approach. Unlike inadvertent injury to the semicircular canals, violation of the cochlea has a much higher risk of hearing loss. The fistula should be covered with fascia and held in place with bone wax or Gelfoam. Injury to the carotid artery is potentially life-threatening. The wall of the petrous carotid artery is usually thinner than the cervical carotid artery and leaving a thin plate of bone over the carotid artery is recommended. Injury

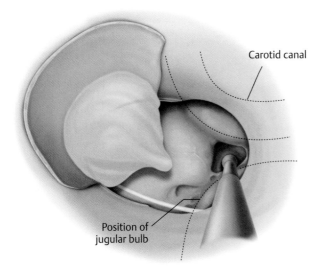

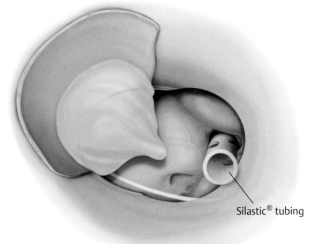

Fig. 4.6 The anterior and inferior bony annulus is removed to give adequate visualization of the hypotympanum. The chorda tympani nerve can be traced inferiorly and posteriorly to identify the facial nerve.

Fig. 4.7 The jugular bulb and carotid artery are identified before more bone is removed medially. Jacobsen's nerve can be followed inferior to identify the jugulocarotid spine.

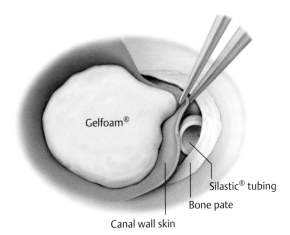

Fig. 4.8 Bone pate is used to repair the hypotympanic defect, and the soft tissue of the external auditory canal is returned to the normal positions.

to the petrous carotid artery should be treated with immediate packing and pressure. Distal control can be achieved with a balloon catheter, and proximal control can be achieved through the neck. Once bleeding has adequately been controlled, the artery can be adequately exposed and repaired with the assistance of a vascular surgeon. Despite successful repair, a cerebral infarct is still a possibility.

◆ Conclusion

Access to the petrous apex is dependent of the location of the lesion and the surrounding vital structures. Using a combination of CT and MRI, most lesions can be characterized without a tissue diagnosis, and appropriate surgical planning will allow successful drainage without morbidity. Most preoperative symptoms can be controlled with good long-term results with adequate surgical drainage.

Suggested Readings
Arriaga MA, Brackmann DE. Differential diagnosis of primary petrous apex lesions. Am J Otol 1991;
    12:470–474 Review. Erratum in: Am J Otol 1992 May;13:297
Brackmann DE, Toh EH. Surgical management of petrous apex cholesterol granulomas. Otol Neurotol
    2002;23:529–533
Fong BP, Brackmann DE, Telischi FF. The long-term follow-up of drainage procedures for petrous apex
    cholesterol granulomas. Arch Otolaryngol Head Neck Surg 1995;121:426–430
Giddings NA, Brackmann DE, Kwartler JA. Transcanal infracochlear approach to the petrous apex. Oto-
    laryngol Head Neck Surg 1991;104:29–36

5

The Retrosigmoid Approach

Jose N. Fayad, Rick A. Friedman, and Marc S. Schwartz

The retrosigmoid approach represents a modification of the classic suboccipital approach. Krause and others first employed the suboccipital route during the latter part of the 19th century. In this procedure, a large bone flap is removed from the suboccipital area, with the anterior limit of the dissection being the first mastoid cell. In the retrosigmoid approach, the anterior limit of the dissection is the sigmoid sinus. Superiorly, bone is removed up to the inferior margin of the transverse sinus. The retrosigmoid approach offers a more favorable angle of view into the cerebellopontine angle (CPA) and a markedly reduced need for cerebellar retraction than does the classic suboccipital approach.

◆ Overview

Modern neurotology began in the early 1960s when William F. House and others began employing the operating microscope in their approach to the contents of the CPA. Over the years, a multitude of approaches have been described and refined to approach lesions and diseases of the CPA and the internal auditory canal (IAC). Now, neurotologists and neurosurgeons have an armamentarium of operative techniques to approach different areas and pathologies of the CPA and skull base. Some of these approaches can be combined to obtain wider exposure and remove tumors involving both posterior and middle fossae. The use of the operating microscope and the development of these approaches have significantly reduced mortality and morbidity in the treatment of CPA lesions.

The retrosigmoid approach offers a panoramic view of the CPA. Indications for the retrosigmoid approach are summarized in **Table 5.1**. The retrosigmoid approach is a hearing-preserving operation that is used for tumors with mainly extracanalicular extension into the CPA and minimal extension into the IAC. Factors affecting hearing preservation in vestibular schwannoma are summarized in **Table 3.2** (p. 29).

◆ Surgical Anatomy

The retrosigmoid approach provides a panoramic view of the posterior fossa from the tentorium to the foramen magnum. Access is provided to the cerebellar hemisphere, the lateral aspect of the pons and medulla, and the root entry zone and cisternal course of cranial nerves V to XI. Although exposure superiorly is limited by the tentorium, this approach could be combined with a middle fossa or transtentorial exposure.

The retrosigmoid craniotomy is based on the transverse and sigmoid sinuses. The precise location and configuration of these structures is relatively variable, so attention to the preoperative imaging is critical. Because the anatomy of the suboccipital

Table 5.1   Indications for the Retrosigmoid Approach
Vestibular schwannoma
Meningioma
Epidermoids
Chondroma
Chondrosarcoma
Chondroblastoma
Chordoma
Trigeminal schwannoma
Infraclinoidal basilar tip aneurysms
Vascular decompression of cranial nerves V, VII, IX, and X
Cranial nerve neurectomies (trigeminal, nervus intermedius, vestibular, and glossopharyngeal nerves)
Vascular disorders of the vertebrobasilar system and parenchymal lesions of the brainstem and the cerebellum

region is not immediately apparent upon external inspection, an ability to visualize the location of these sinuses is important. The transverse sinus lies along a posterior extension of the Frankfurt line. This is also the level of the superior attachment of the suboccipital muscle bulk. The sigmoid sinus typically runs along the posterior edge of the mastoid process.

Although the sigmoid sinuses are co-dominant in about half of all patients, the right sinus is dominant approximately 40% of the time and the left in the remainder. Special care must be taken when working over a dominant sinus, because injury to such a sinus, and subsequent thrombosis, may be catastrophic. In contradiction to the transmastoid approaches, a far-forward sigmoid sinus is an advantage in the retrosigmoid approach. This is typically seen as a result of a contracted mastoid related to chronic mastoid disease during childhood. Preoperative identification of a contracted mastoid may alter the choice of surgical approach in selected cases.

The focal point of this approach is the porus of the internal auditory canal. Access into the canal can be obtained via drilling of its posterior lip. Drilling is limited by the posterior semicircular canal. Five millimeters of canal can be reliably exposed in all cases without injury to the inner ear; in selected cases, up to 10 mm can be exposed.

◆ Surgical Technique

The authors administer preoperative antibiotics and continue them for 24 hours postoperatively. Intraoperative furosemide and mannitol are given to allow easier temporal lobe retraction. We administer dexamethasone intravenously during the procedure and continue this for 24 hours postoperatively. Long-acting muscle relaxants are avoided during surgery so as not to interfere with facial nerve monitoring.

The patient is positioned lateral on the operating table and is carefully secured to allow rotation of the table. The patient's shoulder must be taped down to prevent hindrance of the operative trajectory. A Mayfield headholder is used, and the head is positioned in a relatively neutral position, but with gentle flexion and approximately 10 to 15 degrees of derotation. In patients with large shoulders, the vertex can also be tilted downward. In addition to prepping the scalp, an area of abdomen, flank, and back is also prepped. This is done to allow for both harvesting of abdominal fat for grafting and also intraoperative lumbar puncture, if necessary.

A curved incision is made behind the ear, with its vertex about three finger-breadths behind the ear and its bottom below the tip of the mastoid (**Fig. 5.1**). A scalp flap is raised subcutaneously. This is extended to the periosteum overlying the mastoid. An L-shaped incision is made in the periosteum along the posterior edge of the mastoid and along the superior insertion of the suboccipital muscles (**Fig. 5.2**). The suboccipital muscles are elevated in the subperiosteal plane and are retracted medially and inferiorly. To obtain sufficient exposure, the flap is undermined posteriorly. Also, exposure and elevation of the digastric muscle from its groove is imperative. The suboccipital muscles can be dissected along their fibers to obtain sufficient inferior exposure. Bleeding from the emissary veins is controlled before drilling.

Next, the craniotomy is performed. The craniotomy is based on the posterior aspect of the sigmoid sinus and the inferior aspect of the transverse sinus (**Fig. 5.3**). We utilize cutting and diamond burs to carefully remove bone overlying these structures. Identification of the sigmoid sinus is facilitated by entry into posterior mastoid air cells. The sigmoid sinus can be followed to the transverse-sigmoid junction and then to the transverse sinus. A rectangular craniotomy is performed, with dimensions of approximately 3 cm along the sigmoid sinus and 2.5 cm along the transverse. Care must be taken to avoid avulsing and emissary veins as the flap is removed. These veins must be isolated, coagulated, and divided before the flap is removed. All mastoid air cells are occluded with bone wax.

The dura is opened with a Y-shaped incision with flaps based upon the transverse and sigmoid sinuses (**Fig. 5.4**). In most cases, cerebrospinal fluid (CSF) will drain from over the surface of the cerebellar hemisphere, resulting in brain relaxation. In some cases, and especially those of larger tumors, flow over the cerebellum is impeded. In these cases, drainage of CSF is facilitated by several maneuvers. First, the patient is placed in the reverse-Trendelenburg position. The inferior cerebellar hemisphere is gently retracted over a cottonoid, and, under the operating microscope, the cisterna

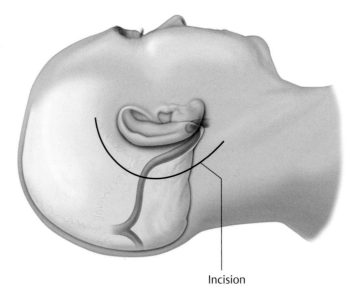

Incision

Fig. 5.1 Postauricular incision.

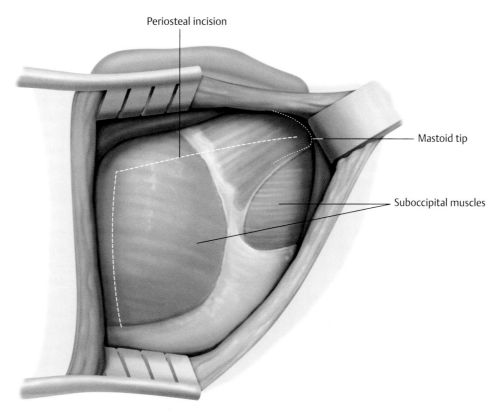

Periosteal incision

Mastoid tip

Suboccipital muscles

Fig. 5.2 Musculoperiosteal flap.

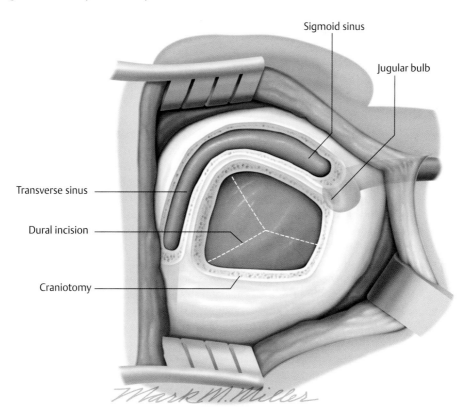

Sigmoid sinus

Jugular bulb

Transverse sinus

Dural incision

Craniotomy

Fig. 5.3 A 3- × 2.5-cm suboccipital craniotomy defect is created just behind the posterior edge of the sigmoid sinus and below the transverse sinus.

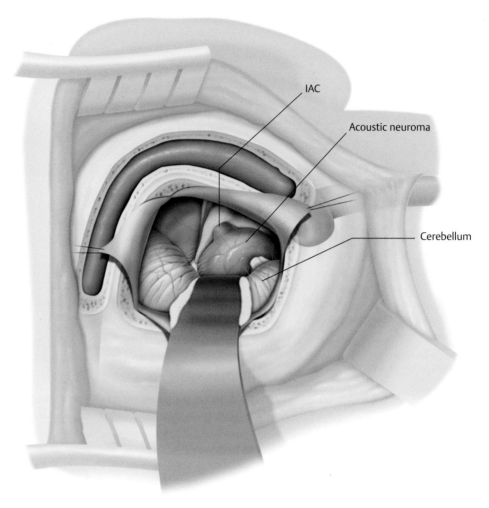

Fig. 5.4   A Y-shaped dural incision. IAC, internal auditory canal.

magna is entered just inferior to the lower cranial nerves. If this dissection is difficult, therapeutic lumbar puncture can be performed. With the drainage of 20 to 30 cc of CSF, the brain relaxes.

To obtain sufficient tumor exposure, the arachnoid overlying the cerebellopontine angle (CPA) is widely opened. Opening is carried from the tentorium to below the lower cranial nerves. Any bridging petrosal veins are carefully coagulated and divided. These maneuvers allow the brain to fall back with gravity, thus exposing the posterior face of the tumor.

Drilling of the posterior lip of the IAC is performed next. The dura is incised over the bony canal. A U-shaped flap is developed by cutting the dura over the porus area and extending the incisions laterally. Bone is removed from the posterior aspect of the canal first to expose the dura of the IAC. Bone is drilled away until the lateral end of the tumor is identified (**Fig. 5.5**). Usually the exposure is limited to the medial two thirds of the IAC. Trying to expose the lateral one third of the canal may result in opening the vestibule or the common crus, causing loss of hearing. Once the exposure of the IAC is completed, the dura overlying the canal is opened. Tumor is exposed, and vestibular fibers are divided at the lateral dome of the tumor. The facial nerve and cochlear nerves are identified. However, dissection of tumor in a lateral to medial direction is avoided to prevent traction on the cochlear nerve (**Fig. 5.6**).

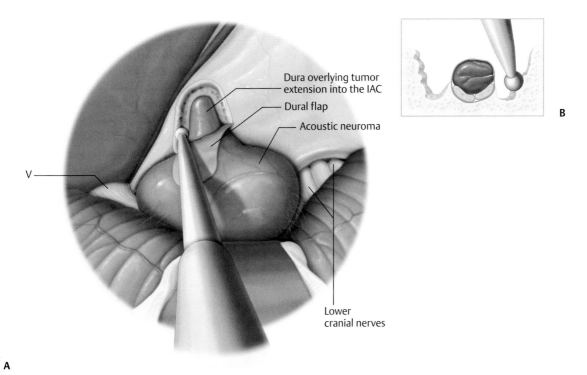

Dura overlying tumor
extension into the IAC

Dural flap

Acoustic neuroma

V

Lower
cranial nerves

A

B

Fig. 5.5 (A,B) IAC drilling.

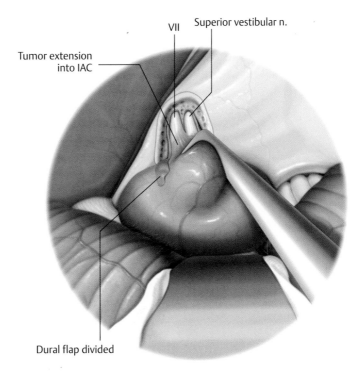

VII   Superior vestibular n.

Tumor extension
into IAC

Dural flap divided

Fig. 5.6   The facial nerve and cochlear nerves are identified.

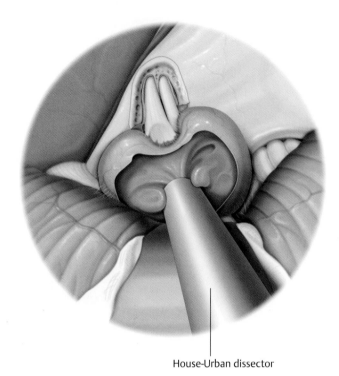

House-Urban dissector

Fig. 5.7 Tumor debulking.

Tumor dissection proceeds with internal debulking **(Fig. 5.7)**. After the tumor is softened, it is separated from the cerebellar hemisphere and any posterior vessels. The eighth nerve root is identified at the brainstem, and tumor is carefully dissected free from all elements of this nerve in a medial to lateral direction. After the tumor has been dissected free from the brainstem, the facial nerve can be identified more anteriorly along the brainstem surface. The courses of these nerves are highly variable, and dissection proceeds accordingly. After additional debulking of tumor, the plane between the tumor and nerves is followed to the porus and into the IAC. Remaining vestibular fibers are divided, and the tumor is removed (**Fig. 5.8**).

After tumor has been removed, hemostasis is obtained. Any air cells that were entered at the IAC are filled with bone wax, and an abdominal fat graft is used to further occlude the flow of CSF in this area. If possible, a single 4–0 suture is used to hold the fat graft in proper position (**Fig. 5.9**). The dura is tacked together, and, because true watertight dural closure is generally impossible, the dural closure is augmented with an onlay collagenous graft. Cranioplasty is performed using titanium mesh. The closure may incorporate the craniotomy flap. This bone flap, however, is usually quite small. Additional abdominal fat is also incorporated into the closure, obliterating any dead space between the dura and the outer table (**Fig. 5.10**).

The scalp is closed in layers. Given the design of the opening, these layers are overlapping. This acts as an additional barrier to CSF egress. Special care is taken at the inferior portion of the wound, as this is the most likely site of any postoperative leakage. A mastoid pressure type dressing is applied and kept in place for 3 days (see Technical Pearls, below).

◆ Limitations

Limitations include a higher incidence of postoperative headaches and CSF leaks. The reason for the higher incidence of headache is unknown, but it is thought to be due to

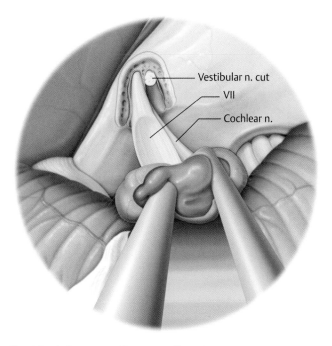

Fig. 5.8 IAC contents after tumor dissection.

soilage of posterior fossa arachnoid by bone dust during intradural drilling of the posterior wall of the IAC. This creates a form of chronic aseptic meningitis that is responsive to steroids. Another explanation for the headaches is adhesion of the posterior fossa dura to the suboccipital musculature. The higher incidence of CSF leaks is explained by the difficulty in sealing all the cells in the petrous apex, especially when it is extensively pneumatized. Another disadvantage is poor exposure of the ventral aspect of the pons and medulla due to the relatively posterior angle of view. The posterior aspect of the clivus is obstructed by the course of cranial nerves V to XI.

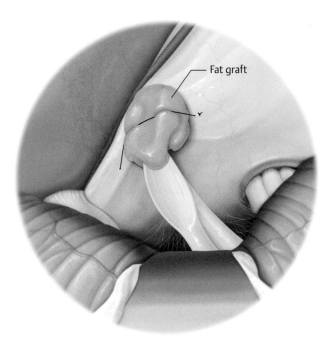

Fig. 5.9 Fat graft or muscle over the IAC.

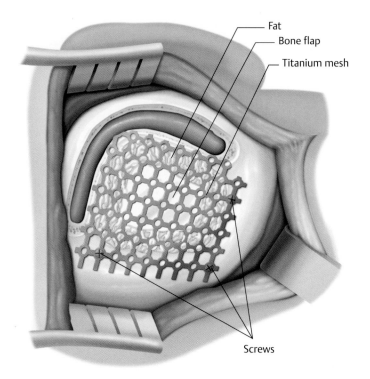

Fat
Bone flap
Titanium mesh

Screws

Fig. 5.10   Closure of bony defect and cranioplasty.

◆ Technical Pearls

- Empty the CPA cistern.
- This approach entails minimal cerebellar retraction.
- Identify the area of the vestibular aqueduct as the most lateral end of dissection in hearing preservation surgery.
- Do not dissect blindly into the IAC.
- Sharply dissect the tumor from medial to lateral.

◆ Conclusion

Advantages of the retrosigmoid approach are wide access of the CPA and the potential for hearing preservation. The retrosigmoid approach is capable of addressing most lesions of the CPA.

Suggested Readings

Cohen NL. Retrosigmoid approach for acoustic tumor removal. Otolaryngol Clin North Am 1992;25:295–310 Review

Lang J Jr, Samii A. Retrosigmoidal approach to the posterior cranial fossa. An anatomical study. Acta Neurochir (Wien) 1991;111:147–153

Tringali S, Ferber-Viart C, Fuchsmann C, Buiret G, Zaouche S, Dubreuil C. Hearing preservation in retrosigmoid approach of small vestibular schwannomas: prognostic value of the degree of internal auditory canal filling. Otol Neurotol 2010;31:1469–1472

6

The Translabyrinthine Approach to the Skull Base

William H. Slattery

The translabyrinthine approach is the most direct approach to the cerebellopontine angle. It was first used by William F. House in the 1960s to remove acoustic tumors, and it resulted in a significant drop in the mortality associated with acoustic tumor removal. The House Clinic has been using this approach since that time. More than 5,000 acoustic tumor (vestibular schwannoma) surgeries using the translabyrinthine approach have been performed at House Clinic. The approach provides excellent exposure to the cerebellopontine angle, allowing early identification of the facial nerve in the labyrinthine segment. The entire facial nerve can be exposed from the brainstem to the stylomastoid foramen. One advantage of this approach is that the entire tumor can be visualized extradurally, reducing the requirement for any type of retraction on the brain. The main disadvantage of the translabyrinthine approach is the sacrifice of hearing. This approach is most commonly used for vestibular schwannoma removal, although it may also be used for total cranial nerve VIII section for disabling vertigo when no useful hearing remains, and for facial nerve tumor removal or facial nerve repair following temporal bone fractures.

The translabyrinthine approach is ideal for vestibular schwannoma removal, regardless of the size of the tumor, when the hearing is poor. It is also useful in tumors larger than 2.0 cm when chances of hearing preservation are extremely poor. The approach has many advantages including minimal cerebellar retraction. The lateral end of the internal auditory canal (IAC) can be dissected to ensure complete tumor removal from this area, and this approach allows consistent visualization of the facial nerve in the labyrinthine section.

Another advantage of the translabyrinthine approach is that the patient is in the supine position with the head turned away from the surgeon, reducing the risk associated with the sitting position of the classic suboccipital approach where the risk of air embolism was significant. The translabyrinthine approach poses no danger of air embolus and does not require retraction of the cerebellum. Most of the surgical approach is extradural, which lessens any trauma to the brain. The tumor can be directly approached and dissection begun without any retraction on the brain. This extradural dissection also decreases the risk of spreading bone dust into the cerebellopontine angle, which may contribute to the headaches associated with the suboccipital procedure.

This approach may be used for tumors other than vestibular schwannomas including meningiomas, cholesteatomas that involve the petrous bone or posterior fossa, cholesterol granulomas in which the hearing has been lost, and glomus tumors. If the facial nerve is lost during tumor removal, a direct nerve anastomosis may be performed. This technique may also be used when a facial nerve schwannoma requires removal. The facial nerve may be removed from the fallopian canal in the vertical and horizontal segments. Mobilization of the facial nerve allows the temporal portion of the facial nerve to be swung down into the cerebellopontine angle for a direct nerve anastomosis. Neuragen tubules can facilitate nerve anastomosis in the cerebellopontine angle,

Table 6.1   Indications
• Large acoustic neuromas
• Acoustic neuromas with poor hearing
• Massive cholesteatomas
• Cerebellopontine angle tumors with poor hearing
• Auditory brainstem implant placement
• Growing acoustic neuromas, status post–radiation treatment

as suturing is difficult due to the lack of epineurium surrounding the facial nerve stump at the brainstem. This offers the best opportunity for facial reanimation with an immediate direct end-to-end nerve anastomosis or, on the rare occasion, an interpositional nerve graft. The disadvantage of the translabyrinthine approach is sacrifice of any residual hearing. Therefore, the procedure is reserved for patients with poor hearing, or patients whose tumor is larger than 2.0 cm in size, in which case hearing preservation is extremely rare.

◆ Indications and Patient Selection

The choice of approach toward a tumor in the cerebellopontine angle is based on tumor type, size, location, and baseline hearing status (**Table 6.1**). Vestibular schwannomas that are large with no serviceable hearing are ideal for this approach. Small tumors that extend no more than 1.0 cm into the cerebellopontine angle with good residual hearing may be removed via a middle fossa approach described in Chapter 3. Vestibular schwannomas that are medial in location with very little projection into the IAC and good residual hearing are usually approached via a retrosigmoid/suboccipital approach. The decision to attempt hearing preservation depends on the status of the preoperative hearing and location of the tumor. Serviceable hearing is defined by the 50/50 rule: this definition requires that the pure-tone average be better than 50 dB and the speech discrimination score be greater than 50%. The status of the contralateral ear must also be taken into consideration when deciding the approach as, rarely, these tumors may present in an only-hearing ear or a better-hearing ear. Vestibular schwannomas larger than 2 cm are usually removed with the translabyrinthine approach, as the chance of preserving the hearing is poor in tumors this large. The choice of approach for meningiomas may be different from that used with vestibular schwannomas, even when located in the same position. Meningiomas have a tendency to displace rather than invade the cochlear and facial nerves, and therefore they have a better chance of hearing preservation, even with large tumors. Therefore, a hearing preservation approach may be selected even if the hearing is poor. Hearing improvement can occur with meningioma resection.

No tumor is too large to be removed via the translabyrinthine approach. Larger tumors require an expanded exposure with more bone removal over the middle fossa and posterior fossa dura. The House Clinic has removed all large acoustic tumors via the translabyrinthine approach for the past 50 years.

◆ Surgical Technique

General endotracheal anesthesia with inhalation agents is used. Muscle relaxants are used only for induction, as they may interfere with nerve monitoring, specifically intraoperative facial nerve monitoring. An oral gastric tube and Foley catheter are placed. Antibiotics with good cerebral spinal fluid penetration are given prior to skin incision. Cefuroxime is our antibiotic of choice in non–penicillin-allergic patients, whereas vancomycin is used in those patients with penicillin allergy. Intravenous antibiotics are given for 24 hours and perioperative steroids are used. The patient is instructed to use Hibiclens solution (Mölnlycke Health Care, Norcross, GA) daily for the 3 days preoperatively to reduce skin bacteria.

The average blood loss with translabyrinthine procedures is less than 250 cc. The need for blood transfusion is extremely rare, but all patients have a type and screen performed preoperatively. One to two units of blood are reserved for patients with large tumors, as the risk for transfusion increases with very large tumors greater than 2.5 cm. Patients are offered the opportunity to directly donate 1 to 2 units of their own blood preoperatively to be available for use during surgery. This has to be done at least 3 to 4 weeks in advance of the surgery. Iron supplements are recommended for these 3 to 4 weeks to increase the hematocrit after donation.

Positioning

The patient is placed in the supine position with the head turned away from the surgeon. The table is rotated 180 degrees so that the foot of the table is next to the anesthesiologist. This allows the anesthesiologist to control the table for movement. The surgeon is seated at the table with the scrub nurse across from the surgeon. The microscope is placed at the head of the table. The head is placed on a donut or a gel pad to prevent pressure necrosis on the contralateral scalp. No fixation of the head is required.

Skin Incision

Hair is shaved from the postauricular and temporal areas. The skin is cleaned with a povidone-iodine (Betadine) solution and a sheet of Ioban is placed over the entire area. Facial nerve monitoring is considered the standard of care for all vestibular schwannoma procedures and all translabyrinthine procedures. The Medtronic (Jacksonville, FL) facial nerve electromyogram (EMG) monitor is recommended, as it has been specifically designed for this use. Needle electrodes are placed in the orbicularis oris and orbicularis oculi muscle (**Fig. 6.1**). A facial nerve EMG is recorded, and this EMG is then used to monitor the facial nerve throughout the case. The lower abdomen is also prepped and draped with Ioban to allow for harvesting of fat graft. The fat graft will be placed in the temporal bone defect after the tumor is removed. The navel is prepped in the abdominal field for orientation. The fat graft is obtained from the left lower quadrant to prevent later mistaking the incision for an appendectomy scar. One percent lidocaine with 1/100,000 epinephrine is injected into the postauricular area. The epinephrine assists with hemostasis.

A postauricular incision is made approximately 3.0 cm behind the auricular sulcus (**Fig. 6.2**). As a general rule a larger tumor requires a more posterior incision. This allows for additional decompression of the dura posterior to the sigmoid sinus. A two-layer incision is created, with the first part of the incision in the skin and the second incision involving the temporalis muscle and periosteum. Ideally, these two incisions should be offset, which helps prevent cerebrospinal fluid (CSF) leakage. The first incision involves the scalp flap just superficial to the temporalis fascia and mastoid periosteum, allowing elevation and anterior movement of the pinna. The second incision is through the periosteum and temporalis muscle, and is T-shaped with the horizontal incision approximately 1.0 cm above the linear temporalis and the vertical incision just posterior to the external ear canal. The Lempert elevator is used to

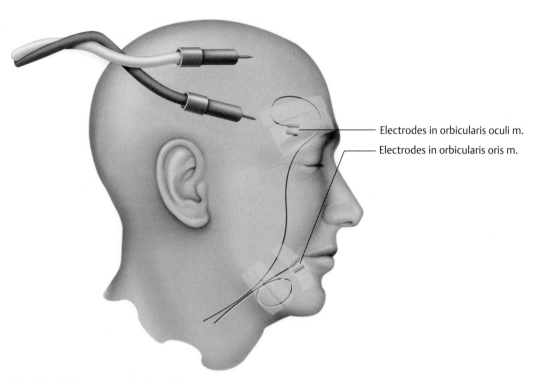

Electrodes in orbicularis oculi m.
Electrodes in orbicularis oris m.

Fig. 6.1   Facial nerve monitoring of face.

elevate the periosteum off the bone of the mastoid. Care must be taken not to tear the skin of the external auditory canal, otherwise a CSF leak may develop posteriorly. The periosteal flap is brought posteriorly, and a large self-retaining retractor is used to retract the tissue, thus exposing the mastoid cortex for extensive bony dissection. Electrocautery may be required to remove the periosteum off the mastoid tip at the

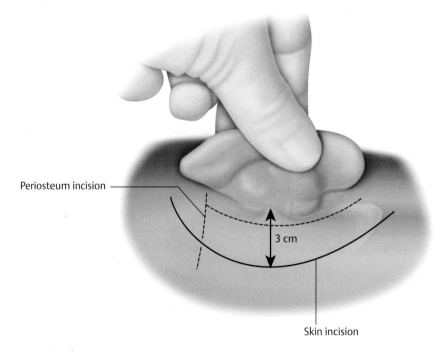

Periosteum incision

3 cm

Skin incision

Fig. 6.2   Skin incision.

insertion of the sternocleidomastoid muscle. Care is taken in elevating the periosteal flaps as the same tissue is needed for closure to aid in prevention of cerebral spinal fluid leaks.

The temporalis muscle is retracted superiorly and the periosteum retracted anteriorly up to the level of the ear canal. At this time, muscle may be harvested for later packing of the eustachian tube and middle ear space, which is performed routinely to prevent CSF leaks. Care should be taken to prevent removal of the temporalis fascia, as the fascia is used to help with closure. Once the soft tissue and periosteum have been elevated, the entire temporal bone should be visualized anteriorly to the external auditory canal, inferiorly to the mastoid tip, and posteriorly to the occiput. The bone over the temporal lobe should also be exposed. The mastoid tip is exposed, although care is required when approaching the anterior mastoid tip as the facial nerve lies in the tympanomastoid fissure. The anterior skin flap and periosteum can be retracted forward with sutures placed into the periosteum. An operative sponge is placed around the auricle to prevent necrosis of the auricle.

Mastoidectomy

A complete cortical mastoidectomy is performed (**Fig. 6.3**). There are two schools of thought on the translabyrinthine approach regarding a mastoidectomy. Some surgeons prefer to leave bone over important structures such as the dura and sigmoid sinus, only to remove this bone after further medial dissection has been performed. This technique can be very useful during training procedures with residents or fellows, because important structures are protected during the drilling. The disadvantage of this approach is that it limits the angle of exposure because the dura cannot be compressed due to the thin shelf of bone left over the dura and sigmoid sinus. My preference is to remove all bone as dissection continues medially, creating a large angle of exposure. A cortical mastoidectomy is performed with a standard T-incision. The first bony cut is along the linear temporalis, with a second cut directly behind the

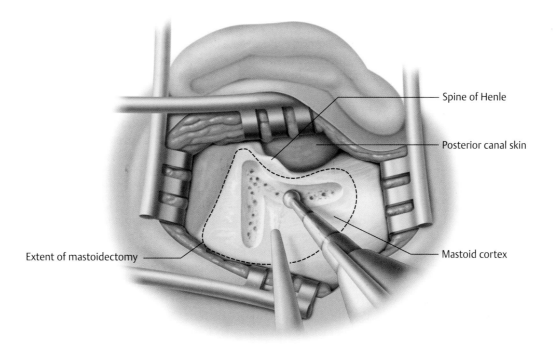

Fig. 6.3 Cortical mastoidectomy.

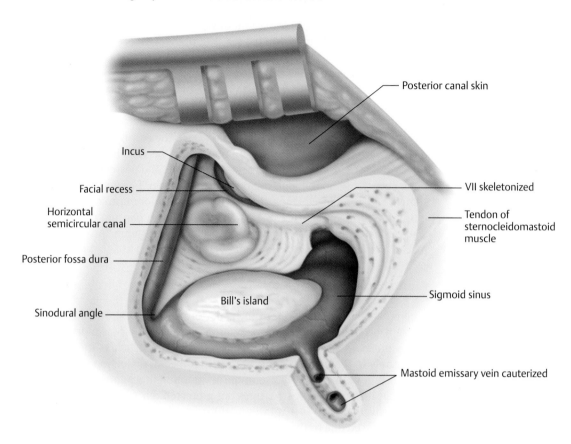

Fig. 6.4   Complete mastoidectomy.

external ear canal. All cortical bone is removed from the mastoid. The middle fossa dural plate and sigmoid sinus are identified. All air cells are removed from behind the external ear canal to identify the external ear canal. Bone is removed down to the mastoid tip for exposure; however, cortical bone is left on the mastoid tip to allow screws to be placed for titanium mesh cranioplasty plating. In contrast to chronic ear disease, it is usually not necessary to remove bone up toward the zygomatic arch. In chronic ear disease the epitympanic space must be opened widely. In contrast, the surgeon rarely needs to remove this bone in a translabyrinthine approach.

It is important that the surgeon performing the translabyrinthine approach be familiar with dissection in the posterior fossa. A criticism of the translabyrinthine approach is that it does not allow adequate exposure and it is difficult for the neurosurgeon to work in such a tight space. This is true only if the translabyrinthine approach is not done correctly. The angle of exposure is important, especially as the surgeon works medially, because the wider the exposure laterally, the more working area that is available for the dissection in the cerebellopontine angle. A very narrow translabyrinthine approach will significantly limit and make dissection much more difficult in the cerebellopontine angle.

Bone is removed off of the middle fossa plate from the sinal dural angle forward to the posterior limit of the external bony ear canal. All air cells are removed from the bony external ear canal so that a thin shelf of bone is all that remains. The sigmoid sinus is identified, and a thin layer of bone ("Bill's island") is left on top of the sigmoid sinus. Bill's island was extremely important when older drills were used as they had a tendency to cut and tear open the sigmoid sinus (**Fig. 6.4**). New high-speed air-driven drills rarely cause this problem, but nonetheless, this acts as a protective factor. Care must be taken in compressing the bone over the sigmoid sinus or compressing the sigmoid sinuses as blood clots can arise. This becomes especially important in patients with bilateral acoustic tumors. Although rarely causing problems, increased cranial pressure can arise postoperatively from an occluded sigmoid sinus.

The mastoid emissary vein has a very consistent anatomic relationship located posteriorly to the midportion of the sigmoid sinus. Bone is removed posteriorly to the sigmoid sinus over the posterior fossa dura for large tumors and in anatomic cases where the sigmoid sinus is found in a more anterior location. Bone may be removed up to 2.0 cm behind the sigmoid sinus. The mastoid emissary vein is removed from the bone and coagulated. Ideally, a diamond drill can be used to drill on each side of the mastoid emissary vein until a small tag is left that is coagulated with a bipolar cautery. It is best to leave a small piece of the mastoid emissary vein next to the sigmoid sinus, which makes cauterization easier.

Upon completion of the cortical mastoidectomy, the middle fossa plate, the sigmoid sinus, and the posterior ear canal have been identified. Bone is removed down to the antrum so that the incus and horizontal semicircular canal may be identified. The horizontal semicircular canal is a landmark, which helps with identification of the facial nerve and labyrinth. The vertical segment of the facial nerve may be identified and skeletonized. Bone should be left over the facial nerve. The retrofacial air cells may be opened, but care must be taken to prevent the drill bit from undercutting into the facial nerve. Air cells are removed down to the digastric ridge, and air cells should also be removed from the mastoid tip. Fat packing is easier when all the air cells have been removed, but this also helps prevent CSF leak. The bone over the sinodural angle should be removed with care, as the superior petrosal sinus lies underneath this area. Occasionally small fragments of bone will embed into the sinus, and removal can cause bleeding. Bipolar cautery will usually control this. If significant bleeding occurs, packing the sinus with Surgicel should control the bleeding. Bone wax is placed over the Surgicel, which prevents the Surgicel from getting caught up in the drill during further dissection.

Labyrinthectomy

The hard bone of the labyrinth may be drilled with a cutting or diamond drill bit, depending on the comfort of the surgeon (**Fig. 6.5A**). More experienced surgeons may use a cutting drill bit, whereas those with less experience are encouraged to use a diamond drill bit. The risk of complications such as facial nerve injury or damage to the dura increases as drilling continues medially. The horizontal semicircular canal should be identified as a result of the mastoidectomy. Safe drilling may be performed superior to the horizontal semicircular canal and posterior to the posterior semicircular canal (**Fig. 6.5B**). This general guideline prevents injury to the facial nerve. Drilling is continued to outline the circular nature of the semicircular canals. The circular nature of the semicircular canal should be retained until all semicircular canals are outlined to help prevent disorientation by the surgeon. Snake eyes is defined as a cut across the semicircular canals when both ends of the canal are facing lateral and the circular orientation has been lost, and this is to be avoided. The horizontal semicircular canal bisects the posterior semicircular canal creating a T-formation. The superior semicircular canal is entirely superior to the horizontal canal, and the common crus is identified as the junction of the posterior and superior semicircular canals. If the incus has been removed, the suction irrigator is positioned over the facial nerve to protect the facial nerve during drilling. Cases have been reported in which the drill rolled over the top of the horizontal semicircular canal, injuring the facial nerve. The first goal of the labyrinthectomy is to have all three semicircular canals

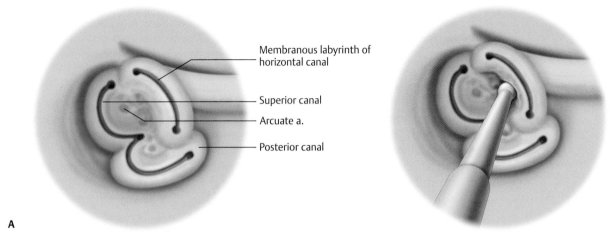

A   B

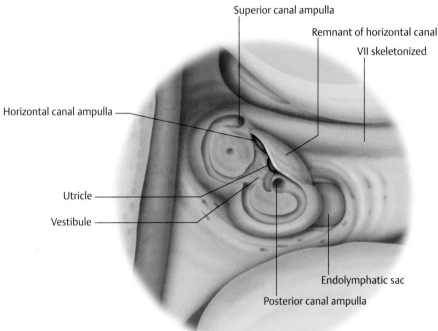

C

Membranous labyrinth of horizontal canal

Superior canal

Arcuate a.

Posterior canal

Superior canal ampulla

Remnant of horizontal canal

VII skeletonized

Horizontal canal ampulla

Utricle

Vestibule

Endolymphatic sac

Posterior canal ampulla

Fig. 6.5 Labyrinthectomy. **(A)** The orientation of the labyrinth; **(B)** drilling performed superior to the horizontal semicircular canal; **(C)** labyrinthectomy completed with the vestibular open.

completely outlined so that the anatomic relationships remain intact. The superior semicircular canal is opened to the ampulla and vestibule. The junction of the ampulla and vestibule is a landmark that identifies the superior aspect of the IAC. The ampulla of the posterior canal is a landmark for the inferior border of the IAC. The posterior semicircular canal is also opened into the vestibule. The inferior bony removal is to the level of the jugular bulb. Bone is removed medial to the jugular bulb and in many cases anterior to the jugular bulb. In cases of a high jugular bulb, bipolar cautery may be used on the dura overlying the jugular bulb to allow the jugular bulb to shrink.

The endolymphatic sac, or the superior aspect of the endolymphatic sac, is located at the midportion of the posterior semicircular canal. The endolymphatic sac must be cut away from the dura to complete bony dissection. The endolymphatic sac may be followed into the vestibule along the endolymphatic duct. The vestibule is opened widely once the remaining labyrinthectomy has been performed (**Fig. 6.5C**).

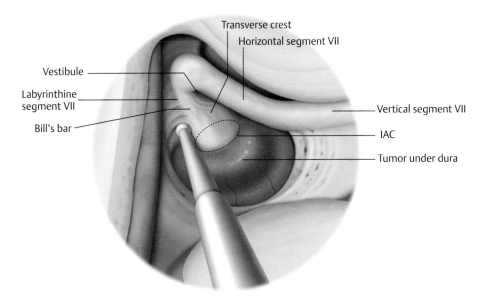

Fig. 6.6 Facial nerve identification.

Once the labyrinthectomy is completed and the vestibule is opened, the surgeon is ready to proceed with facial nerve decompression and identification of the IAC.

Facial Nerve Identification

It is helpful to perform facial nerve decompression after the labyrinthectomy has been performed. The facial nerve is identified in its entirety from the IAC and is skeletonized throughout the mastoid just proximal to the stylomastoid foramen (**Fig. 6.6**). A large diamond drill bit can be used at this time to complete the labyrinthectomy along the horizontal semicircular canal, identifying the facial nerve. The use of large diamond drill bits helps reduce the possibility of injury to the facial nerve. The side of the diamond drill bit is used as opposed to the end, which also reduces potential hazard to the nerve. The facial nerve is identified and traced along the second genu into the vertical segment. The ideal situation is to leave a thin layer of bone over the facial nerve and not leave the facial nerve exposed in any area of the temporal bone. The large diamond drill bit allows this to be accomplished very quickly. The vestibule is opened up completely. A large amount of bone is usually found over the second genu. Inexperienced surgeons often leave a large amount of bone in this area, thus limiting the exposure. Care must be taken to prevent undercutting of the facial nerve with a drill bit, as damage can occur in this area. The stapedius muscle is frequently encountered medial to the vertical segment of the facial nerve. The retrofacial air cells are explored once the vertical facial nerve has been identified. The sigmoid sinus is followed down to the jugular bulb. Bone marrow may frequently be encountered in the retrofacial air cells. If excessive bleeding occurs, bone wax is used to control this.

Drilling is continued along the horizontal portion of the facial nerve until the geniculate ganglion is exposed. The labyrinthine segment of the facial nerve is then traced just anterior to the ampulla of the superior semicircular canal. As the facial nerve is skeletonized, the cribriform area of the superior vestibular nerve entering the vestibule will be seen posterior to the labyrinthine facial nerve. Bone overlying the labyrinthine segment of the facial nerve will be removed, but this is done after the IAC has been skeletonized.

Middle Ear and Eustachian Tube Plugging

Plugging of the eustachian tube and obliteration of the middle ear with muscle have been routine in our practice for the past several years. This reduces the risk of cerebral spinal fluid rhinorrhea through the eustachian tube. Once the labyrinthectomy has been completed and the facial nerve identified, the area of the middle ear is accessed through the facial recess approach or through the antrum, which has already been exposed. The incus is removed and the tensor tympani muscle is cut. Care must be taken not to injure the tympanic membrane. Iodine is left in the external ear canal during the prep, so if injury to the tympanic membrane occurs, iodine will be seen. Usually, three small pieces of thick Surgicel are packed down the eustachian tube orifice. The anesthesiologist should be alerted when this technique is being performed, as occasional stimulation along the fifth cranial nerve may result in increased blood pressure. Previously harvested muscle is then packed into the middle ear filling the entire middle ear space. It is advisable to do this prior to tumor dissection so a blood clot can form with the muscle, creating a fibrin seal around the muscle plug in the middle ear space.

Internal Auditory Canal

Identification of the IAC remains one of the more difficult aspects of the translabyrinthine approach. The superior aspect of the IAC is identified by the ampulla of the superior semicircular canal. This portion of the superior canal identifies the area where the superior vestibular nerve exits the lateral end of the IAC and, as described earlier, is just posterior to the labyrinthine segment of the facial nerve. Similarly, the singular nerve exits the IAC at the posterior semicircular canal ampulla, and the inferior vestibular nerve exits the IAC into the saccule. The IAC is just medial to the vestibule structures. Identification of these structures helps delineate the superior and inferior aspect of the IAC.

Once the vestibule has been identified, drilling should be performed in a superior to inferior fashion to identify the most posterior aspect of the IAC. An eggshell thickness of bone is left over the dura of the IAC to avoid injury to the underlying structures until all of the bony dissection has been completed. Large tumors that expand the IAC may distort this anatomy. As the posterior aspect of the IAC is identified, drilling is performed medially until the junction between the posterior fossa dura and IAC is encountered. It is important to remember that the IAC is directed anteriorly, or away from, the surgeon as drilling is completed from a lateral to medial direction.

Once the IAC is identified from the posterior fossa dura to the vestibule, drilling is performed inferiorly. The superior aspect of the IAC is the last area to be exposed because the facial nerve lies in this vicinity. It is better to have more landmarks identified prior to drilling near the facial nerve located within the IAC. The jugular bulb may require skeletonization. A thin layer of bone typically remains over the jugular bulb. Drilling is continued anteriorly until the cochlear aqueduct is encountered. The cochlear aqueduct, once opened, allows CSF to drain from the posterior fossa. The cochlear aqueduct is the inferior and anterior limit of the dissection. Inferior to the cochlear aqueduct lie the lower cranial nerves just underneath the dura. Drilling below this area may result in injury to cranial nerves IX, X, and XI. In cases of a high jugular bulb, drilling continues in front of the jugular bulb by positioning the surgeon's hands more superiorly. Decompression of the middle fossa plate can really assist the surgeon with the proper angle. The IAC is skeletonized along its entire length until the anterior portion of the canal is reached. The goal of drilling is to have a 270-degree exposure of the IAC. It is recommended that bone be removed along the posterior fossa dura anterior to the IAC to allow adequate exposure of the tumor. The dura may need to be reflected inferiorly to have exposure anterior to the IAC, especially with large tumors that extend in this direction. This inferior/anterior exposure can assist with the identification of the lower cranial nerves once the dura is opened.

After the inferior dissection has been completed with the cochlear aqueduct identified, bone is removed around the posterior aspect of the IAC to the porus acusticus until the entire inferior lip of the IAC is removed. Diamond drill bits may be used for this part of the dissection. At this time, the bone of the posterior fossa dura has been removed inferiorly along the sigmoid sinus to the jugular bulb, reaching to the cochlear aqueduct and slightly anterior to this. The inferior portion of the section is now complete, and superior dissection above the internal auditory is now performed. Bone dissection above the IAC is performed last due to the presence of the facial nerve in this location. It is important to have all landmarks identified prior to attempting the identification of the facial nerve in the labyrinthine canal. Often the facial nerve will lie just beneath the bone in the anterior superior location, and heat from the drill can cause damage to the facial nerve, resulting in neurapraxia. The drill bit must not touch the facial nerve or tear the dura in this location as that may also result in injury. At this time, bone should have been removed from the posterior and inferior aspect of the IAC. Drilling is continued into the anterior petrous apex above the IAC. In many cases there are air cells in this area that can be opened. Temporal bones that have extensive aeration will have air cells into the anterior petrous apex that must be waxed to prevent later CSF leakage. The superior aspect of the IAC must be fully identified, and drilling is continued until the anterior border of the IAC is identified. If the inferior anterior border has been identified, this can be used as an approximation for the anterior superior border and width of the canal. Drilling is continued superior to the IAC, again medially to expose the entire IAC. A thin shelf of bone is usually left in this area to be removed after drilling is completed. The lateral end of the IAC is left until last, as this is the most dangerous area with regard to damage to the facial nerve. It is extremely important that all bone is removed from the superior aspect all the way to the anterior border of the IAC. Otherwise, dissection of the facial nerve will be more difficult. Drilling is continued along the posterior fossa dura superior and anterior to the IAC, into the anterior petrous apex. This allows easier exposure into the posterior fossa dura, especially when facial nerve dissection is being performed.

The lateral end of the IAC is the last area to be exposed (**Fig. 6.7**). The facial nerve canal is separated from the superior vestibular canal by a vertical crest termed "Bill's bar." Upon exiting the IAC the facial nerve travels slightly superior, and care must be taken to prevent damage to the facial nerve in this location. Removal of bone superior to this area allows easier dissection. Occasionally, the middle fossa dura will be low hanging, requiring dural elevation for the labyrinthine segment to be exposed. The entire labyrinthine segment of the facial nerve is typically drilled out to allow decompression of the facial nerve in this area. Small fragments of bone may be removed, allowing only the dura to cover the nerve. Copious irrigation should be performed to prevent the drill from causing heat damage to the facial nerve. At this time, all bone is removed from the underlying dura. Irrigation to remove all bone dust is performed. The entire approach has been performed extradurally with no retraction to the brain structures.

Intradural Dissection

After all bone and bone dust has been removed, the dura is opened, exposing the tumor. The dura over the IAC is opened first. An incision is created laterally near the inferior vestibular nerve (**Fig. 6.8**). This can be done with a right-angle hook. Once the dura has been opened, sharp scissors may be used to cut the dura directly posteriorly. This cut is from lateral to medial. Occasionally, a large vessel may run under the dura near the porus acusticus, and care must be taken to prevent injury to this vessel. The posterior fossa dura is also opened at this time. An incision just anterior to the

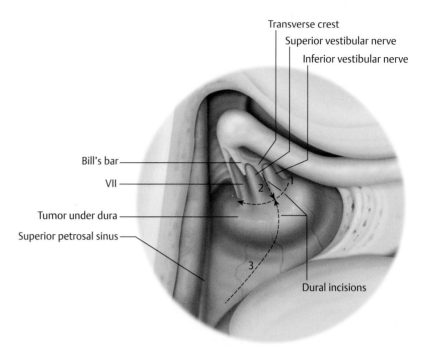

Fig. 6.7   Internal auditory canal nerves in the lateral end of the IAC. 1, Incision around the internal auditory canal; 2, incision opening the interior auditory canal; 3, posterior fossa dura incision.

junction of the superior petrosal sinus and sigmoid sinus is created. This cut is first made with a sharp knife, and then the dura is retracted laterally to allow direct visualization of the medial side of the dura. The dura is then cut directly toward the IAC. Cottonoid may be placed over the cerebellum and the tumor. The dura is then re-

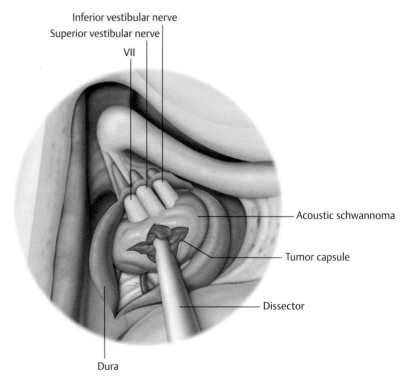

Fig. 6.8   Dural opening.

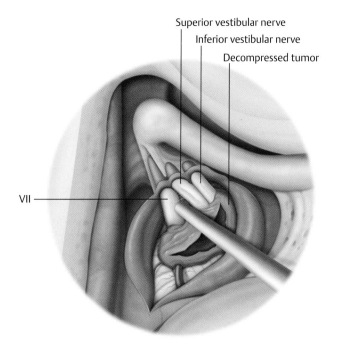

Superior vestibular nerve

Inferior vestibular nerve

Decompressed tumor

VII

Fig. 6.9 Tumor dissection.

flected both anteriorly and inferiorly. Occasionally, sutures may be required to re-tract the dura, although if all bone is removed the dura will usually open and stay retracted. Occasionally, relaxing incisions must be made along the superior and infe-rior aspect of the porus acusticus. Care is taken in connecting the posterior fossa inci-sion with the incision over the IAC, as a vessel as described above may be found in this location.

The dura is reflected inferiorly to expose the inferior aspect of the dissection. The entire inferior dissection is exposed. The dura overlying the superior aspect of the IAC is then retracted, with care taken as one approaches the anterior IAC where the facial nerve is located. The dura must also be separated from the superior vestibular nerve and then along Bill's bar to the labyrinthine segment (**Fig. 6.9**). It is best to do this with a sharp dissection, and typically it is performed with a sharp right-angle hook. The labyrinthine facial nerve is identified throughout the labyrinthine segment. The dura may be reflected from atop of the IAC, allowing complete exposure of the facial nerve. The facial nerve stimulator may be used at this time to positively identify the facial nerve. The facial nerve stimulator is set at the 0.05-mA stimulation level. This usually results in a very robust response on the facial nerve monitor. After the dura is opened, the petrosal vein is found lying up underneath the superior petrosal sinus. Care must be taken in reflecting the dura, as occasionally large blood vessels may enter into the petrosal veins near the tumor. Cottonoids may be placed posteriorly over the cerebellum, and then between the cerebellum and the tumor. This defines the posterior dissection for the tumor. The cistern may be drained inferiorly by open-ing arachnoid bands to allow further CSF release, thereby relaxing the entire intra-cranial contents.

The lateral end of the IAC is now approached. The vertical crest, or Bill's bar, is iden-tified, and the superior vestibular nerve is posterior to this crest. The superior ves-tibular nerve is removed posteriorly after stimulation with the facial nerve monitor correctly identifies that there is no stimulation of the superior vestibular nerve and positive stimulation of the facial nerve. The superior vestibular nerve is retracted posteriorly, which allows a plane to be developed between the superior vestibular

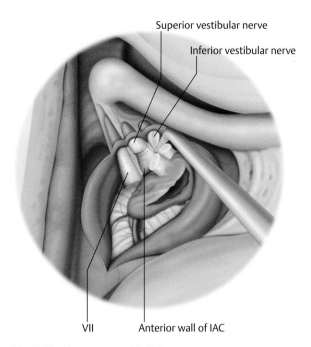

Superior vestibular nerve

Inferior vestibular nerve

VII   Anterior wall of IAC

Fig. 6.10   Tumor removal in IAC.

nerve and the facial nerve. Acoustic tumors usually arise from the superior vestibular nerve and, in this case, there is a potential space called the facial nerve plane. With superior vestibular tumors, the plane is between the tumor and facial nerve. If the tumor involves the inferior vestibular nerve, then the superior vestibular nerve is still dissected away from the facial nerve as this correctly creates a plane between the facial nerve and the tumor. The plane between the facial nerve and superior vestibular nerve or tumor is usually easily identified within the IAC and can be followed medially until the area of the porus acusticus is identified. At this time, the facial nerve usually becomes much more adherent to the tumor and it also thins out. The long fine right-angle hook is usually used to identify the superior vestibular nerve and the facial nerve canal. The nerve hook can be placed until it hits the vertical crest along the superior vestibular nerve canal. The hook can then rise over the crest to correctly identify the labyrinthine facial nerve. The hook can be placed under the superior vestibular nerve to withdraw it from the superior vestibular nerve canal. Early and positive identification of the facial nerve within the labyrinthine facial canal is one of the advantages of the translabyrinthine approach.

The inferior vestibular nerve and cochlear nerve may be cut at this time in small tumors to allow complete retraction of the tumor away from the facial nerve (**Fig. 6.10**). In large tumors the adherence of the inferior vestibular and cochlear nerve can prevent traction along the facial nerve that may occur during large tumor dissection. Therefore, we usually identify the facial nerve and then debulk and remove a significant amount of the tumor before the lateral end of the IAC is completely dissected. The cochlear and inferior vestibular nerves are cut to allow complete removal of tumor contents within the IAC.

Vestibular Schwannoma Tumor Removal

The translabyrinthine approach is most commonly used for vestibular schwannoma removal. We use this approach to remove tumors in which the hearing has been lost, or large tumors of any size when hearing preservation is unlikely. Once the facial nerve has been identified and CSF pressure released, the tumor edges are identified. The posterior aspect of the tumor is separated from the cerebellum. Cottonoids are placed in this plane. As dissection occurs around the tumor, cottonoids are placed to prevent damage to critical structures that may have been separated by earlier dissection. The lower cranial nerves are separated from the tumor. In large tumors the lower cranial nerves may be stretched and be very adherent to the tumors, so cottonoids are placed over the lower cranial nerves to protect them during tumor dissection. A fenestrated neurotologic suction tip is useful to avoid suction traction to delicate nervous tissue. This type of device has holes in the side, which prevent significant suction of neuro-tissue up into the suction that may cause damage to this tissue. Cranial nerve V is identified superiorly, and small cottonoids are used to develop a plane between it and the tumor. At this time, the tumor's anterior is gutted. The surface of the tumor is carefully inspected to ensure there is no nervous tissue in this area. Bipolar cautery is used on any vessel. The facial nerve stimulator may be used on a high setting such as 3 mA to confirm that the facial nerve is not located anywhere near the dissection. An opening is created through the tumor capsule. A House-Urban or ultrasonic dissector is used to gut the interior of the tumor. As the interior of the tumor is gutted or removed, the capsule of the tumor can fall in upon itself. A specimen must be obtained and sent to pathology for confirmation of the schwannoma. The surface of the capsule is followed as gutting is completed. This is followed posteriorly to the brainstem. Care must be taken during manipulation and dissection around cranial nerves V, IX, and X, as changes in heart rate and blood pressure may occur. The anesthesiologist is notified when dissection is being performed around the structures. If a change in vital signs occurs, then dissection is briefly halted until vital signs return to normal.

Large vessels may be found around the tumor. Care is taken to separate these vessels from the tumor capsule. Perforating vessels that extend into the tumor are taken with bipolar cautery. Dissection is performed to try to expose as much of the perforating vessels as possible so that a small stump may be left on the originating vessel. The facial nerve may be located once the brainstem is identified. The tumor must be rotated laterally near the brainstem to allow identification of the facial nerve. There are small venus plexus over the root entry zone of the facial nerve, and care must be taken during dissection of this area. Cranial nerve VIII is usually identified posterior to the facial nerve. This must be cut prior to dissection of the facial nerve to allow adequate visualization of the facial nerve at the brain stem. Usually the facial nerve is identified prior to cutting the stump of cranial nerve VIII. The tumor is rotated superiorly or inferiorly depending on the direction of the facial nerve. The plane along the brainstem can usually be easily dissected, although there may be quite a few adhesions in large tumors between the facial nerve and the tumor capsule. Ideally, we try to rotate the tumor posteriorly and inferiorly to avoid stretching the facial nerve. Once the bulk of the tumor has been removed, the facial nerve usually can be dissected from the remaining portion of the tumor. The entire dissection along the facial nerve is performed with direct visualization. If there is any question of the direction of the facial nerve, the facial nerve stimulator is used to stimulate the nerve and trace its location. The facial nerve direction can be quite variable, although the nerve is usually superior and anterior to the tumor. Sharp dissection is performed along the course of the facial nerve, with care taken not to stretch the facial nerve during separation of the nerve from the tumor (**Fig. 6.11**).

Once the tumor is completely removed, bacitracin irrigation is used to rinse the wound and reduce the chance of infection. Bacitracin irrigation may also be used toward the end of drilling and is attached to the suction irrigator, although it is usually done when diamond drill bits are being used. Bacitracin irrigation can create foam that makes suction difficult. Bacitracin irrigation, along with intravenous preoperative antibiotics, has reduced the risk of meningitis.

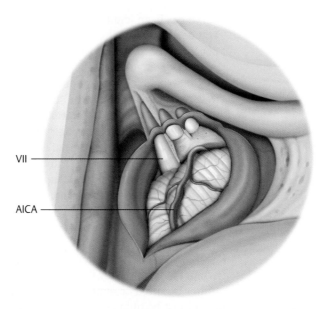

VII

AICA

Fig. 6.11 Tumor out, facial nerve intact. AICA, anterior inferior cerebellar artery.

Closure and Cranioplasty

After total tumor removal, the dura is closed, the mastoid defect is obliterated with fat, and a titanium mesh cranioplasty is performed (**Figs. 6.12 and 6.13**). The wound is copiously irrigated with bacitracin solution to remove any blood clots. The cottonoids are removed and the irrigation makes this easier. The posterior fossa defect is filled with irrigation solution, and this is observed for several minutes to ensure that no additional bleeding is going to occur. It is best to control bleeding at this time prior to dural closure, allowing extra time to identify any bleeding and correct it. Bipolar cautery is used on any actively bleeding vessels. Gelfoam soaked with thrombin can be used for small oozing vessels that may be found on the brainstem.

Abdominal fat is obtained from the left lower abdomen. The dead space from the fat removal is closed with deep sutures to reduce the risk of abdominal wound hematoma. The wound is closed with a layer of Vicryl sutures, and a Penrose drain is inserted in the surgical cavity to help prevent hematoma formation. Steri-Strips are placed across the incision. The fat is cut into strips and soaked in bacitracin irrigation during the procedure. Typically, the fat is obtained earlier, prior to tumor removal, and is left to soak in bacitracin irrigation solution. We keep this covered to prevent contamination.

The posterior fossa dura is reapproximated and 4–0 nylon is used to hold this together. If the dura can be preserved, then a fairly good reapproximation of the dura can be performed. In some cases the dura is very thin and tears, and the suture must be used as a scaffolding to support the fat (**Fig. 6.12**). Rarely the dura of the IAC is preserved, but if it is, the superior portion can be placed over the facial nerve. In some instances where a large dural defect may exist over the posterior fossa, a piece of temporalis fascia or Duragen may be laid across the posterior fossa dura. The fat is cut into long strips approximately 4.0 cm in length by 1.0 cm in width. The strips of fat are inserted through the dural defect and then superior and inferior to the IAC. The fat is layered into the defect and tightly packed between the external ear canal, middle ear space, and posterior fossa dura. Care is taken not to put pressure on the facial nerve in the labyrinthine segment during packing of the fat. The facial nerve monitor is watched very closely during this time for any signs of irritation to the facial nerve due to excess fat packing.

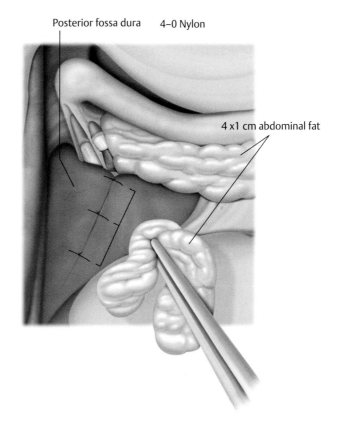

Fig. 6.12 Dural closure and fat packing.

A titanium mesh cranioplasty is performed once the mastoid cavity is filled with fat (**Fig. 6.13**). Titanium mesh is cut to the appropriate size and fixed to the cranium using four microscrews. A translabyrinthine plate specifically designed for translabyrinthine surgery has been created and is available, which makes cutting the titanium mesh no longer necessary. Typically, the periosteum in the overlying muscle layer is

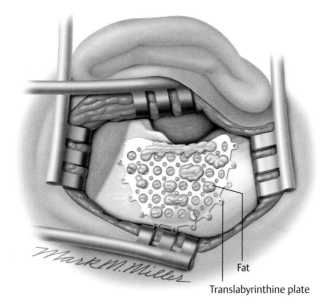

Fig. 6.13 Cranioplasty.

retracted superiorly and posteriorly to expose the bone surrounding the mastoid opening. The titanium, once in place and reconstructed to the lateral surface of the mastoid, does not impinge on the posterior skin of the external auditory canal. The plate reconstructs the surface of the cranium at the same time it applies pressure over the fat, keeping the fat in position and preventing it from coming loose. This technique of titanium mesh cranioplasty has significantly reduced the risk of CSF leakage following translabyrinthine procedure. The rate of CSF leakage at our institution after translabyrinthine procedure is now 3.3% using the new method of titanium mesh closure. This compares with rates of 10.9% and 8.7% in previous series in which other methods of closure were used. The rate of CSF leakage requiring reoperation is 0.5% compared with 2.5% in our old series. Thus, we recommend titanium mesh cranioplasty for all translabyrinthine procedures, as this has statistically reduced the rate of CSF leaks following translabyrinthine removal of tumors. The wound is closed in layers, with the periosteal flaps being closed first and the skin flap closed second. Steri-Strips are applied to the scalp incision, and the head dressing is applied.

◆ Postoperative Care

Immediately after surgery the patients are transferred to the intensive care unit where they will stay with continuous monitoring for the first 24 hours after surgery. The typical hospital stay is 3 to 5 days. The abdominal wound is changed on the first postoperative day and the Penrose drain removed. A light dressing is placed on the wound. Steroids are continued for the first 7 days postoperatively. Antibiotics are continued for 24 hours. The mastoid dressing stays in place for 3 days postoperatively, and Steri-Strips are removed from the incision 7 to 10 days postoperatively. Progressive ambulation begins after surgery. The patient is encouraged to sit up and begin oral intake the first postoperative day. A progressive ambulation occurs while in the hospital with the assistance of physical therapy. Early ambulation can reduce the risk of deep vein thrombosis and pulmonary embolus. Compression boots are continued throughout the postoperative stay until the patient is fully ambulatory.

Observation of clear rhinorrhea or incision swelling is an indication of cerebral spinal fluid leakage. The need for pressure dressings has been significantly reduced following titanium mesh cranioplasty. Vital signs and neurologic checks are frequently performed while the patient is in the hospital to identify any early complications associated with craniotomy. The patient is instructed not to lift or strain for the first 2 weeks following surgery. Vestibular exercises begin at the 2-week postoperative check and continue until the patient has no further dizziness. A postoperative magnetic resonance imaging (MRI) scan is scheduled for 1 year after surgery.

◆ House Clinic Translabyrinthine Results

We recently reviewed 512 patients undergoing primary translabyrinthine at the House Clinic for treatment of a spontaneous unilateral vestibular schwannoma during a 5-year period from 2000 through 2004. This represented 46% of the 1116 patients who underwent treatment for vestibular schwannomas at our practice during that time period. The average tumor size was 2.4 cm, ranging from 0.5 to 5.0 cm. The average age was 49 years, with a range from 13 to 85 years. Anatomic preservation of the facial nerve was obtained in 97.5% of patients. **Table 6.2** demonstrates the relationship between tumor size and facial nerve function. Tumor size significantly impacts the outcome of facial nerve function, with smaller tumors having better results, and tumors larger than 3.5 cm having significantly more risk for postoperative facial nerve paralysis. Total tumor removal was accomplished in 94.5% of patients, and only

Table 6.2 Tumor Size and Facial Function at 1 Year

HB Grade	Number of Patients (%)				
	<1.5 cm	**1.5–2.5 cm**	**>2.5–3.5 cm**	**>3.5 cm**	**All Sizes**
I	68 (86)	122 (71)	61 (58)	14 (39)	265 (68)
II	4 (5)	20 (12)	23 (22)	5 (14)	52 (13)
III	2 (3)	13 (8)	11 (10)	6 (17)	32 (8)
IV	5 (6)	13 (8)	5 (5)	5 (14)	28 (7)
V	0 (0)	1 (1)	0 (0)	2 (6)	3 (0.8)
VI	0 (0)	3 (2)	5 (5)	4 (11)	12 (3)
Total	79	172	105	36	392

HB, House Brackmann Facial Nerve Scale

Source: From Brackmann DE, Cullen RD, Fisher LM. Facial nerve function after translabyrinthine vestibular schwannoma surgery. Otolaryngol Head Neck Surg 2007;136:773–777. Reprinted by permission.

a small capsule of the tumor was left in 1.6% patients due to tumor invasion of the facial nerve.

◆ Complications

The translabyrinthine approach remains a very safe and effective method for removal of vestibular schwannomas of any size; however, complications with intracranial procedures may exist. There have been no deaths in our recent series of translabyrinthine approaches. The facial nerve function was preserved in the majority of patients. CSF leak rates have been reduced to 3.3% with titanium cranioplasty. CSF leaks can usually be managed with conservative measures such as lumbar drainage and pressure dressing or over-sewing of the incision. Rarely, a return to the operating room is required for closure of the CSF leak.

Postoperative bleeding with hematoma formation in the cerebellopontine angle is a potentially fatal complication in the early postoperative period. This may present with neurologic changes when the patient loses consciousness and has nonresponsive pupils. An emergency computed tomography (CT) scan can diagnose this condition. The patient is taken back to surgery and the hematoma evacuated. In a recent series, there were four subdural hematomas (0.8%) and three cerebral cerebellopontine angle clots (**Table 6.3**). The risk of infarct, or stroke, is approximately 1%. This is associated with larger tumors. Meningitis occurred in three patients (0.6%). The incidence of meningitis has decreased with the bacitracin irrigation and reduced surgical time. Prophylactic antibiotics have also helped prevent meningitis. Aggressive postoperative treatment when symptoms of meningitis occur such as stiff neck or fever can reduce the sequelae for meningitis. A spinal tap is performed on any patient presenting with symptoms of meningitis. If the white blood count is high, protein is elevated, and glucose reduced, then intravenous antibiotics are started until cultures can dictate the appropriate antibiotic regimen.

◆ Conclusion

The translabyrinthine approach to the cerebellopontine angle provides an excellent approach for acoustic tumors and other lesions of the cerebellopontine angle. This

Table 6.3   Complications

Complication	N	%
CSF leak	28	5.5%
Infarct	5	1.0%
Subdural hematoma	4	0.8%
Meningitis	3	0.6%
Cerebellopontine angle clot	3	0.4%
Hydrocephalus	2	0.4%
Deep vein thrombosis	2	0.4%
Abdominal hematoma	1	0.2%

approach is ideal for large acoustic tumors and other tumors in which hearing preservation is unlikely.

Suggested Readings

Brackmann DE, Cullen RD, Fisher LM. Facial nerve function after translabyrinthine vestibular schwannoma surgery. Otolaryngol Head Neck Surg 2007;136:773–777

Fayad JN, Schwartz MS, Slattery WH, Brackmann DE. Prevention and treatment of cerebrospinal fluid leak after translabyrinthine acoustic tumor removal. Otol Neurotol 2007;28:387–390

House WF. Translabyrinthine approach. In: House WF, Luetje CM, eds. Acoustic Tumors, Vol 2: Management. Baltimore: University Park Press, 1979:43–87

House WH. Monograph. Transtemporal bone microsurgical removal of acoustic neurons. Arch Otolaryngol Head Neck Surg 1964;80:598–757

7

The Transcochlear Approach to Cerebellopontine Angle and Clivus Lesions

Antonio De la Cruz, Karen Borne Teufert, and Jose N. Fayad

The transcochlear approach is the most direct surgical route to midline intracranial lesions arising from the clivus, and to cerebellopontine angle masses arising anterior to the internal auditory canal. These lesions may extend around the vertebrobasilar arteries, and, because traditional surgical approaches were limited by the cerebellum and the brainstem, these lesions had been considered inoperable by many surgeons up to the 1970s. The transcochlear approach does not have these limitations and was designed primarily for meningiomas arising from the petroclinoid ridge, intradural clivus lesions, chordomas, congenital petrous apex cholesteatomas, and primary intradural epidermoids anterior to the internal auditory canal.

◆ Overview

The transcochlear approach evolved to gain access to the base and blood supply of near-midline and midline tumors. Total removal of these lesions through a traditional suboccipital approach is often impossible because of the interposition of the cerebellum and the brainstem. The transpalatal-transclival approach was attempted for these intradural midline lesions, with little or no success. The exposure through the anterior midline is often inadequate; the field is far from the surgeon; the blood supply is lateral, away from the surgeon's view; and intracranial complications due to oral contamination can occur. The retrolabyrinthine approach is limited in its forward extension by the posterior semicircular canal. Tumor access with the translabyrinthine approach is limited anteriorly by the facial nerve, which impedes removal of the tumor's base of implantation, which is anterior to the internal auditory canal, around the intrapetrous carotid artery, or anterior to the brainstem. The development of the extended middle fossa approach and combined transpetrous approach enables complete removal of petroclinoid meningiomas, and is used in patients with useful hearing. The primary limitation with this approach is poor access to tumors with inferior or midline extension.

The transcochlear approach was developed by William F. House and William E. Hitselberger in the early 1970s as an anterior extension of the translabyrinthine approach. It involves rerouting of the facial nerve posteriorly and removal of the cochlea and petrous bone, exposing the intrapetrous internal carotid artery. This approach affords wide intradural exposure of the anterior cerebellopontine angle, cranial nerves V, VII, VIII, IX, X, and XI, both sixth cranial nerves, the clivus, and the basilar and vertebral arteries, without using brain retractors. The contralateral cranial nerves and the opposite cerebellopontine angle are also visible. This wide exposure affords removal of the tumor base and its arterial blood supply from the internal carotid artery.

Table 7.1   Indications for the Transcochlear Approach

Petroclinoid ridge meningiomas

Intradural clivus lesions

Chordomas

Congenital petrous apex cholesteatomas

Primary intradural epidermis anterior to internal auditory canal

In addition, excision and closure of the external auditory canal, as advocated by Brackmann, further increases the anterior exposure for lesions of the petroclival regions and prepontine cistern. Pellet and associates described the widened transcochlear approach for large tumors of the jugular foramen with intrapetrous, intracranial, and infratemporal extensions.

This approach requires no cerebellar or temporal lobe retraction. Exposure and dissection of the petrous apex and clivus beyond the midline allows complete removal of the tumor, its base of implantation, and its blood supply. This is of particular importance in meningiomas. Careful handling and constant monitoring of the facial nerve during rerouting prevents injury to the intratemporal portion of the nerve. However, meningiomas often invade the nerve, and cholesteatomas tend to wrap themselves around it. If the facial nerve is lost during tumor removal, we recommend immediate repair by end-to-end anastomosis or nerve graft interposition. The indications for the transcochlear approach are summarized in **Table 7.1**.

The main disadvantages of this approach are sacrifice of residual hearing in the operated ear and risk of temporary facial palsy. This technique is used when no serviceable hearing exists in the involved ear or when the tumor is too far anterior for the extended middle fossa craniotomy approach or transpetrous approach. With the use of continuous facial nerve monitoring, the incidence of permanent facial nerve paralysis is low. Risks and complications in the immediate postoperative period include transient vertigo, complete hearing loss, and temporary paresis of cranial nerves VII, IX, X, XI, and XII, as well as infection, bleeding, swallowing difficulties, aspiration pneumonia, cerebrovascular accidents, and death.

◆ Surgical Anatomy

Intracranial structures that may be exposed by the classic transcochlear approach include the entire lateral aspect of the pons and upper medulla, cranial nerves V through XI, as well as the midbasilar artery. Its posterior fossa exposure is extensive except inferiorly, where it is limited in the area of the jugular foramen and foramen magnum. The degree to which the neural compartment of the jugular foramen is visible depends on the height of the jugular bulb. Modifications to the transcochlear approach permit identification of the anterior aspect of the pons and both sixth nerves, and improved identification of the basilar artery and vertebrobasilar junction.

◆ Surgical Technique

A wide mastoidectomy and labyrinthectomy are performed, exposing the internal auditory canal. When first described by House and Hitselberger in 1976, the external canal was not removed and only the facial recess was opened to permit anterior exposure. Brackmann modified the approach by removing the entire tympanic mem-

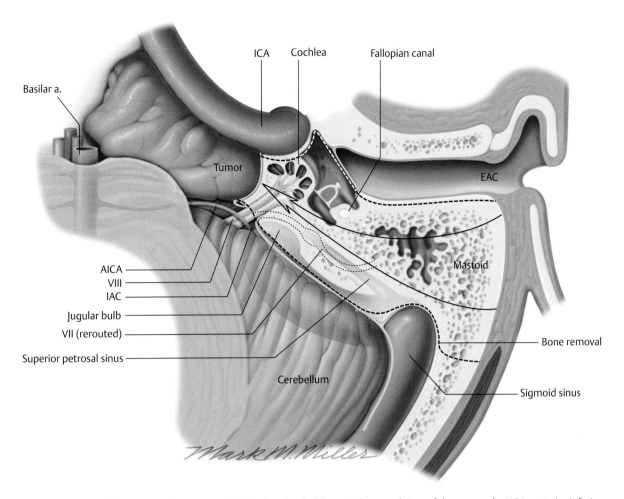

Fig. 7.1 Transcochlear approach: exposure obtained at the skull base at the completion of the approach. AICA, anterior inferior cerebellar artery; EAC, external auditory canal; IAC, internal auditory canal; ICA, internal carotid artery; VIII, eigth cranial nerve; VII, facial nerve.

brane, malleus, incus, and stapes, and performing a blind-sac closure of the external auditory canal, after Fisch.

The facial nerve is completely skeletonized, with transection of the greater superficial petrosal and chorda tympani nerves, and it is rerouted posteriorly out of the fallopian canal. The fallopian canal and the cochlea are completely drilled out, and the internal carotid artery is skeletonized (**Fig. 7.1**). A large triangular window is created into the skull base. Its superior boundary is the superior petrosal sinus; inferiorly, it extends below and medial to the inferior petrosal sinus into the clivus. Anteriorly is the region of the intrapetrous internal carotid artery, and the apex of the triangle is just beneath Meckel's cave. When the dura is opened, this window gives excellent access to the midline without the need for brain retraction. After tumor removal, the dura is reapproximated with dural silk, the eustachian tube is packed with Surgicel and muscle, and abdominal fat is used to fill the dura and mastoidectomy defects and to cushion the facial nerve.

Setup

General endotracheal anesthesia is administered with direct arterial blood pressure monitoring, and a urinary catheter and a nasogastric tube are inserted. Long-acting muscle relaxants are avoided. Intraoperative nerve monitoring is used in all cases.

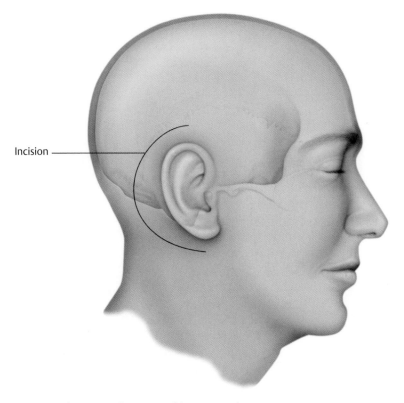

Incision —

Fig. 7.2   Skin incision for transcochlear approach.

Anesthesia is kept light so that changes in blood pressure and pulse brought about by tumor manipulation are not masked. Prophylactic third-generation cephalosporin antibiotics and steroids are used routinely before the skin incision is made. Venous antiembolism compression boots are placed on the patient's legs before the procedure begins.

The patient is placed supine on the operating room table, with the head turned to the opposite side, and is maintained in a natural position without fixation. This position avoids air embolization, minimizes surgeon fatigue, and allows stabilization of the surgeon's hands during the microsurgical procedure.

Incision

A postauricular suboccipital incision is made 5 cm behind the postauricular fold, starting 1 cm above the ear, extending through the occipital bone, and ending at the level of the mastoid tip (**Fig. 7.2**). *This incision can easily be extended inferiorly into the neck to provide control of the great vessels and of the lower cranial nerves, if necessary.* The scalp flap is lifted anteriorly, uncovering the temporalis fascia. The periosteum is incised just above the linea temporalis from the zygomatic root anteriorly to a level posterior to the sigmoid sinus. A second periosteal incision perpendicular to the previous one is carried inferiorly in the direction of the mastoid tip. The periosteal flap is elevated forward to the spine of Henle and to the level of the external auditory canal. The skin of the external auditory canal is initially left in place. In some cases of far anterior-placed lesions, removal of the external auditory canal is necessary. In this case the skin, tympanic membrane, and malleus are removed, and the meatus is closed in three layers (**Fig. 7.3**).

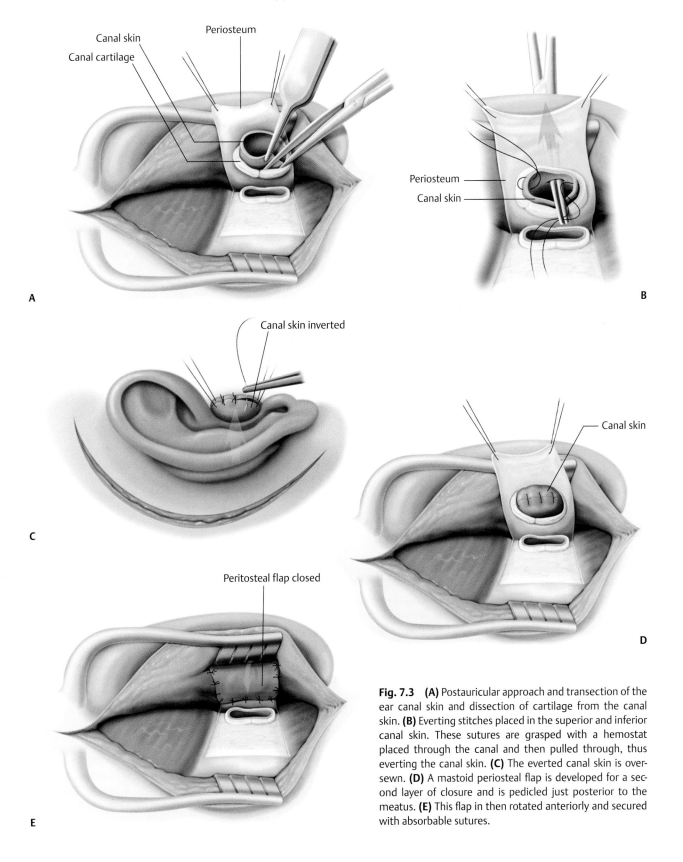

Fig. 7.3 **(A)** Postauricular approach and transection of the ear canal skin and dissection of cartilage from the canal skin. **(B)** Everting stitches placed in the superior and inferior canal skin. These sutures are grasped with a hemostat placed through the canal and then pulled through, thus everting the canal skin. **(C)** The everted canal skin is oversewn. **(D)** A mastoid periosteal flap is developed for a second layer of closure and is pedicled just posterior to the meatus. **(E)** This flap in then rotated anteriorly and secured with absorbable sutures.

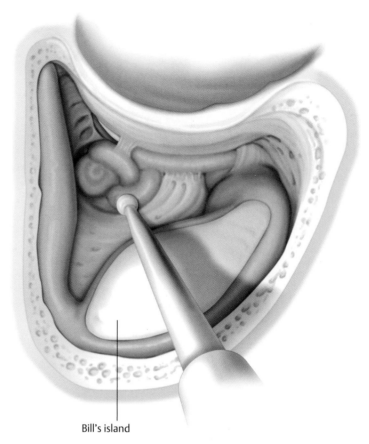

Bill's island

Fig. 7.4 Transcochlear approach: mastoidectomy. There is wide exposure of the posterior and middle fossa dura, with identification of the bony labyrinth and skeletonization of the sigmoid sinus, preserving Bill's island over the dome.

Mastoidectomy

An extended mastoidectomy (**Fig. 7.4**) is performed with microsurgical cutting and diamond burs and continuous suction-irrigation. Bone removal is started along two lines: one along the linea temporalis and another tangential to the external canal. The sigmoid sinus is identified. The mastoid antrum is opened, and the lateral semicircular canal is identified. The lateral semicircular canal is the most reliable landmark in the temporal bone and allows the dissection to proceed toward delineating the vertical fallopian canal and the osseous labyrinth.

The opening of the mastoid cavity is extended posterior to the sigmoid sinus, exposing 1 to 2 cm of suboccipital dura. The larger the tumor, the further back the posterior fossa dura is exposed, to a maximum of 2 to 3 cm. Mastoid emissary veins are dissected, and bleeding is controlled using bipolar cautery and Surgicel packing. Removal of bone over the sigmoid sinus is performed with diamond burs, and an island of bone (Bill's island) may be left over the dome of the sinus initially. This eggshell of bone protects the sinus from being injured by the shaft of the bur. Bone is removed from the sinodural angle along the superior petrosal sinus. The mastoid air cells are exenterated from the sinodural angle, thereby skeletonizing the dura of the posterior and the middle fossae.

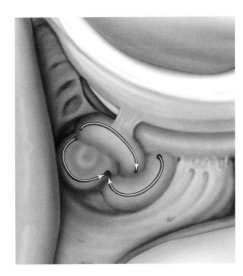

Fig. 7.5 Transcochlear approach: exposure of the internal auditory canal (IAC), skeletonization of the facial nerve from the IAC to the stylomastoid foramen, and extended facial recess. The labyrinthectomy has been completed.

Labyrinthectomy and Exposure of the Internal Auditory Canal

Dissection of the perilabyrinthine cells down to the lateral semicircular canal is completed (**Fig. 7.5**). The facial nerve is identified in its vertical portion between the non-ampullated end of the lateral semicircular canal and the stylomastoid foramen. At this stage, exposing the perineurium of the nerve is not necessary, but it should be clearly and unmistakably identified in its vertical course.

The lateral semicircular canal is fenestrated superiorly, and the membranous portion is identified and followed anteriorly to its ampullated end and posteriorly to the posterior semicircular canal. All three semicircular canals are removed, and the saccule and utricle in the vestibule are identified and removed.

The dissection proceeds along the sinodural angle and the superior petrosal sinus. The dura of the posterior fossa is exposed anteriorly. The jugular bulb is skeletonized and the cochlear aqueduct is also removed. To obtain better control of the lower cranial nerves and the vertebrobasilar junction, the jugular bulb is completely exposed and, if needed, compressed. The internal auditory canal is skeletonized, beginning inferiorly and then around the porus acusticus (**Fig. 7.6**). The falciform crest (transverse) and vertical crest (Bill's bar) are used as identifying landmarks for the facial nerve, and superior and inferior vestibular nerves. The bone of Bill's island over the sigmoid sinus is removed.

Facial Nerve Rerouting (Figs. 7.7 and 7.8)

After removal of the incus, an extended facial recess opening is created. The facial nerve is completely skeletonized from the internal auditory canal to the stylomastoid foramen, including the geniculate ganglion, with diamond burs. Approximately 180 degrees of the fallopian canal bone is removed to facilitate its mobilization. The greater superficial petrosal nerve is cut at its origin near the geniculate ganglion. *The nerve is then reflected posteriorly out of the fallopian canal, with care taken to avoid traction on the nerve, especially near the mastoid genu, which is the site of several*

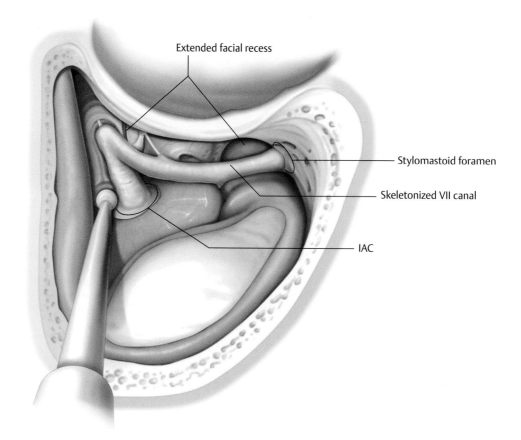

Fig. 7.6 Skeletonization of the jugular bulb and the internal auditory canal (IAC).

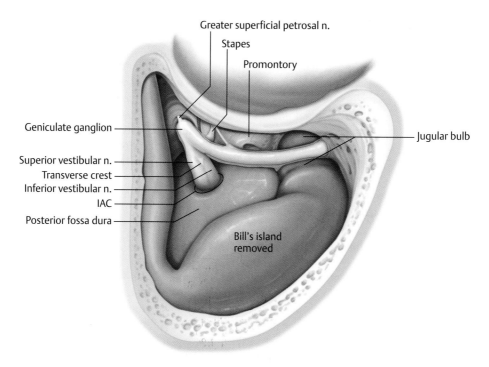

Fig. 7.7 Transcochlear approach: bone over the facial nerve is removed. At this point, the greater superficial petrosal nerve is sectioned. IAC, internal auditory canal.

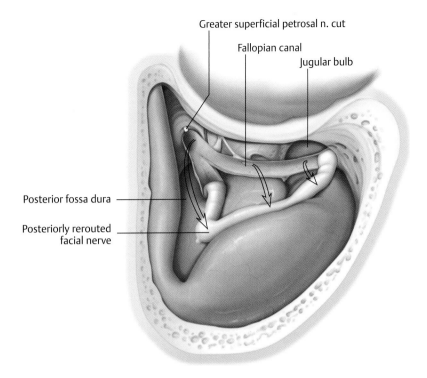

Fig. 7.8 Transcochlear approach: location of the facial nerve after it is completely reflected posteriorly out of the bony fallopian canal.

branches to the stapedius muscle. Care is also taken to avoid kinking of the nerve at the stylomastoid foramen when reflecting it posteriorly. The facial nerve is protected at all times and kept wet.

Closure of the External Auditory Canal (Fig. 7.3)

When further anterior exposure is required, removal and closure of the external auditory canal are also performed. The canal skin is transected at the bony-cartilaginous junction and is undermined laterally. Extra cartilage is removed, and the skin is closed with interrupted nylon sutures in a dimple-like fashion at the external auditory meatus. A flap of mastoid periosteum is developed on a pedicle just posterior to the external auditory canal. This flap is then rotated anteriorly and secured as a second layer of closure for the meatus. After removal of all of the canal skin, the tympanic membrane, and the malleus and incus, the bony external auditory canal is drilled out and excised circumferentially. The eustachian tube is curetted and the packed with Surgicel and temporalis muscle. Care is taken to avoid entering the glenoid fossa.

Transcochlear Drill-Out (Fig. 7.9)

The Fallopian canal and the ossicles have been removed and the promontory is now exposed. Starting with the basal coil, the cochlea is completely drilled out. Bone removal is carried forward around the internal carotid artery, and inferiorly the bone removal extends to the inferior petrosal sinus and jugular bulb. Superiorly, the superior petrosal sinus is followed to Meckel's cave. Medially, bone removal extends to the clivus. At this stage, a large triangular window, covered by dura, has been created into midline of the skull base. Its boundaries are, superiorly, the superior petrosal sinus; inferiorly, below and medial to the inferior petrosal sinus into the clivus; anteriorly,

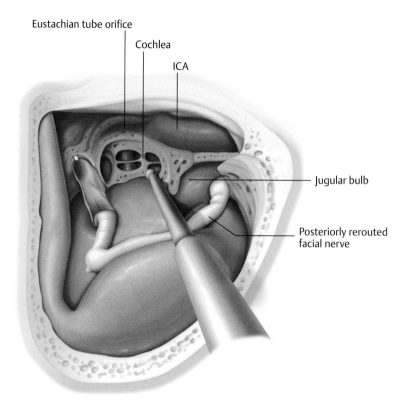

Fig. 7.9   Transcochlear approach: cochlear drill-out. ICA, internal carotid artery.

the region of the internal carotid artery; and medially, the lateral clivus. The apex of the triangle is just beneath Meckel's cave.

Tumor Exposure and Removal (Figs. 7.10 and 7.11)

With meningiomas, arterial feeder vessels from the internal carotid artery were encountered and eliminated during the approach. The diamond bur is used to obliterate these vessels and the base of implantation at the petroclival area. The dura is opened anterior to the internal auditory canal, and the opening is extended as far forward as is necessary for complete tumor exposure. The dural opening extends from the superior petrosal sinus superiorly to the inferior petrosal sinus inferiorly.

The facial nerve is kept on the posterior surface of the tumor. The junction of the intracranial portion of the facial nerve and the skeletonized intratemporal portion is now identified. The nerve is protected and kept moist.

The tumor pseudocapsule is opened, and the center of the main mass of the tumor is removed with the House-Urban rotatory dissector. As the dissection proceeds forward and medially, the basilar artery and cranial nerves IV and VI are identified anterosuperiorly. The vertebral artery appears posteroinferiorly. The tumor is removed from these vessels and their major tributaries under direct vision. In tumors extending across the midline, the basilar artery and its major branches can be dissected posteriorly off the tumor capsule. When the lesion is removed in this fashion, the cranial nerves and the internal auditory canal in the opposite cerebellopontine angle come into view (**Fig. 7.12**). No brain retractors are needed to allow for this exposure.

For dumbbell-shaped tumors, the tentorium can be opened to excise the portion of the tumor that is lying in the middle fossa. Care is taken not to injure the vein of Labbé or the fourth cranial nerve at the edge of the tentorium.

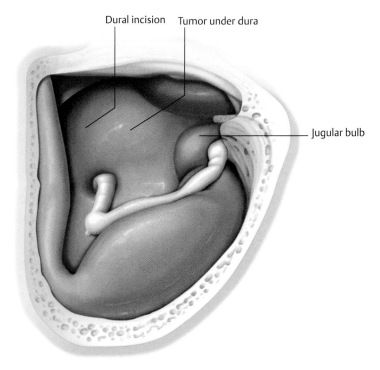

Fig. 7.10 Transcochlear approach: tumor exposure.

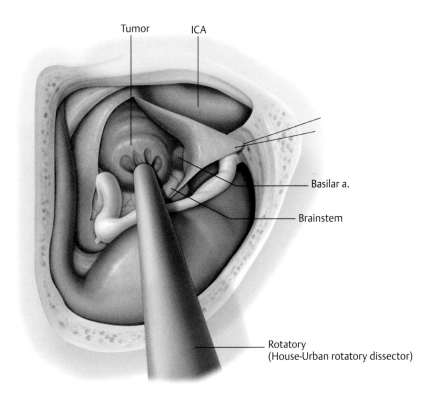

Fig. 7.11 Transcochlear approach: tumor removal.

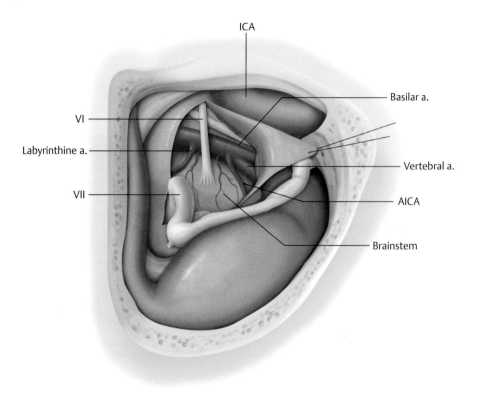

Fig. 7.12 Transcochlear approach: tumor removed. AICA, anterior inferior cerebellar artery; ICA, internal carotid artery.

Closure

After the tumor has been removed, hemostasis is secured. The dura is reapproximated, and the facial nerve is reflected forward. The eustachian tube orifice is plugged with Surgicel, bone wax, and bone pate. Abdominal fat strips are used to fill the dural defect, the mastoid, and skull base defect, as well as to form a bed for the facial nerve. A titanium mesh cranioplasty is performed. The postauricular incision is closed in three layers, and a compressive dressing is placed securely about the head. Lumbar drainage may be indicated for 5 days (see Technical Pearls, below).

◆ Postoperative Care

The patient is observed in the intensive care unit for 48 hours after surgery and remains in the hospital for 5 days. Steroids are continued for 48 hours. Antibiotics are routinely used during the perioperative period. Early mobilization and ambulation allow for avoidance of thromboembolism and recovery from dysequilibrium.

◆ Limitations

The main limitations of this approach are sacrifice of residual hearing in the operated ear and risk of permanent facial dysfunction. With this approach, recurrence is rare when all visible tumor has been removed. Patients with recurrences do not present typically and may have vague complaints of unsteadiness or trigeminal symptoms several years after the initial resection. Annual follow-up with gadolinium-enhanced and fat-suppression magnetic resonance imaging (MRI) is necessary. In cases of suspected tumor regrowth or recurrence, complete reevaluation is performed, and removal or radiation of the recurrent tumor may be recommended.

◆ Technical Pearls

- Inferior extension of incision provides control of great vessels and lower cranial nerves.
- Opening of the mastoid cavity is extended posterior to the sigmoid sinus, exposing 1 to 2 cm of suboccipital dura.
- Falciform and vertical crests are identifying landmarks for the facial nerve and the superior and inferior vestibular nerves.
- Avoid traction on the facial nerve, especially near the mastoid genu.
- For dumbbell-shaped tumors, care is taken not to injure the vein of Labbé or cranial nerve IV at the edge of the tentorium.

◆ Conclusion

Access to midline intradural lesions, intradural petroclival tumors, and cerebellopontine angle tumors arising anterior to the internal auditory canal has traditionally been difficult. With the transcochlear approach, the facial nerve is mobilized, the cochlea removed, and the petrous apex dissected around the internal auditory artery, allowing direct exposure of these lesions and of midline and contralateral cerebellopontine angle structures, without using retraction. Total removal of the tumor and its base and blood supply is possible with this approach. The transcochlear approach is recommended for these lesions in patients with poor hearing. Its safety and efficacy encourage its use.

Suggested Readings

Angeli SI, De la Cruz A, Hitselberger W. The transcochlear approach revisited. Otol Neurotol 2001;22: 690–695

De la Cruz A, Teufert KB. Transcochlear approach to cerebellopontine angle and clivus lesions: indications, results, and complications. Otol Neurotol 2009;30:373–380

House WF. Transcochlear approach to the petrous apex and clivus. Trans Sect Otolaryngol Am Acad Ophthalmol Otolaryngol 1977;84:ORL927–ORL931

Pellet W, Cannoni M, Pech A. The widened transcochlear approach to jugular foramen tumors. J Neurosurg 1988;69:887–894

Sanna M, Mazzoni A, Saleh EA, Taibah AK, Russo A. Lateral approaches to the median skull base through the petrous bone: the system of the modified transcochlear approach. J Laryngol Otol 1994;108: 1036–1044

8

The Combined Petrosal Approach to the Petroclival Region

Rick A. Friedman, Marc S. Schwartz, and Eric P. Wilkinson

The petroclival region represents one of the most difficult anatomic areas to approach surgically. Complex vascular and neural anatomy contributes to the technical difficulty of this region. Historically, several variations of approaches to this region have been used, including traditional neurosurgical pterional and suboccipital routes. Lateral skull base approaches have the advantage of decreasing the operative distance to the tumor and adjacent structures while improving the deep "line of sight" and avoiding excessive brain retraction. The combined petrosal approach to the petroclival region allows for these technical improvements. This approach may be customized based on preoperative hearing thresholds, size of the tumor to be extirpated, and age and condition of the patient.

◆ Overview

Tumors in the petroclival region often extend into both the middle and posterior cranial fossae. Frequently, because of their location, combined petrosal approaches coupling both a middle fossa approach (i.e., the "anterior" portion of the approach) with a presigmoid posterior fossa approach provide the widest and most direct access to these tumors. The terminology in the literature varies, as many authors have applied different names to the particular exposures that they prefer.

The anterior approach preferred at our center is the extended middle fossa approach. This approach is typically combined with a selected posterior fossa approach. In patients with smaller lesions and good hearing, we prefer the retrolabyrinthine approach (retrolabyrinthine presigmoidal transtentorial approach). In larger tumors, a partial labyrinthectomy (also termed "transcrusal") approach may be employed. In very large tumors or in patients in whom hearing conservation is not an issue, a translabyrinthine, transotic (without facial nerve mobilization), or transcochlear approach (with posterior mobilization of the facial nerve) may be employed. These approaches remove more bone to increase visualization and improve the angle of approach to the lesion, while keeping brain retraction to a minimum and decreasing the working distance. When the posterior wall of the external auditory canal (EAC) is removed as is done in the transotic or transcochlear techniques, removal of all EAC skin and the tympanic membrane is performed, and oversewing (modified Rambo closure) of the external auditory canal is required.

Table 8.1   Indications for the Combined Petrosal Approach

Petroclival meningioma

Basilar artery aneurysms

Meckel's cave lesions, including trigeminal schwannoma

Chondroma

Chondrosarcoma

Chondroblastoma

Chordoma

◆ Indications

The combined petrosal approach is utilized to access extensive lesions of the petroclival region. Lesions best accessed via this approach have their origins at the petrous apex, the tentorium, and Meckel's cave. Petroclival meningiomas are the typically approached in this way. Other clival lesions may also be accessed (**Table 8.1**). Petroclival tumors that predominantly involve the prepontine cisternal area anterior to the internal auditory canal (IAC) may be approached with an extended middle cranial fossa approach (see Chapter 3). Lesions that extend posterior to the IAC require the addition of a retrolabyrinthine or translabyrinthine addition, depending on the patient's preoperative hearing. For lesions that extend to the lower clivus/foramen magnum area, the posterior approach may include a far lateral exposure.

◆ Preoperative Workup

Surgical preparation is similar to that for the middle cranial fossa approach. Perioperative antibiotics are administered for 24 hours. Dexamethasone is administered as prophylaxis against edema. Mannitol and furosemide are administered to relax the brain parenchyma and facilitate retraction. Hyperventilation is used as needed. We utilize a Mayfield headholder and rigidly immobilize the patient's head rotated approximately 45 degrees opposite the side of the lesion. It is important not to over-rotate to avoid interruption of venous return via the jugular veins. Exposure and temporal lobe elevation may be facilitated by tilting the vertex slightly downward. Facial nerve monitoring as well as intraoperative auditory brainstem response (ABR) monitoring are regularly employed. Monitoring of additional cranial nerves may be added as indicated.

◆ Surgical Anatomy

Because the petroclival region is a small anatomic area with a large number of critical neurovascular structures, great care must be taken to avoid undue morbidity. The surgeon must be intimately familiar with the anatomy of the region, including the anterior and posterior cranial arterial circulation; the location of the cranial nerves, particularly IV through VIII; the venous drainage patterns of the temporal lobe including the vein of Labbé and other potential temporal bridging veins; and the anatomy of the semicircular canals and fallopian canal.

A key difference between the combined petrosal approach and other approaches to the lateral skull base is the sectioning of the tentorium cerebelli. The tentorium cerebelli is the fold of dura that forms a roof over the posterior cranial fossa, except in the anteromedial region where it forms the incisura. Several main pitfalls pertain to the variations in anatomy that can occur in the dural folds of this region, as well as in the venous drainage pattern variations that accompany them. These are discussed further below.

◆ Surgical Technique

Skin and Soft Tissue Dissection

The skin incision begins just posterior to the anterior hairline in the right fronto-parietal area, and extends approximately superior and posterior to the auricle. The incision is then curved inferiorly, passing posterior to the mastoid region, and ending posterior and inferior to the mastoid tip over the region of the sternocleidomastoid muscle (**Fig. 8.1**). Alternatively, the anterior limb of the skin incision may be extended inferiorly, in the preauricular area.

The skin flap is then sharply elevated and retracted anteriorly and inferiorly. Skin clips are typically not used. Dissection anteriorly is taken down to the superficial layer of the deep temporal fascia, elevating the superficial temporal fascia (temporoparietal fascia) with the skin flap to protect the frontal branch of the facial nerve. After subgaleal elevation of the scalp, deep tissue is raised in several layers. The periosteum of the mastoid and along the inferior temporal line is incised, and the suboccipital muscles are elevated medially and inferiorly. The temporalis fascia is incised just below the superior temporal line, and the posterior portion of the temporalis is elevated anteriorly. The entire mastoid is exposed to the digastric groove posteroinfe-

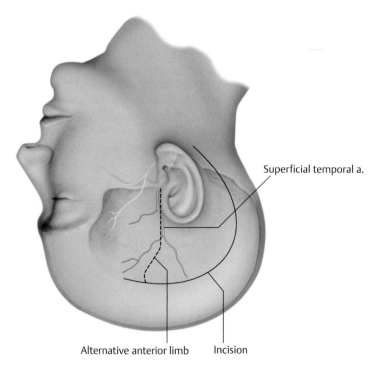

Superficial temporal a.

Alternative anterior limb   Incision

Fig. 8.1 Skin incision. Dashed line shows an alternative to the extension to the frontal area. Superficial temporal artery position is demonstrated.

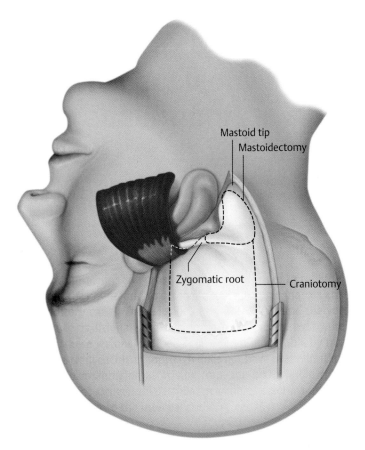

Fig. 8.2 Outline of the posterior and superior craniotomies with the temporalis muscle reflected inferiorly. The superficial temporal artery is preserved, and temporoparietal fascia can be used as a vascularized flap at the time of closure as needed.

riorly and the root of the zygoma anterosuperiorly (**Fig. 8.2**). Sutures or rubber band hooks are used to retract the skin and muscle flaps.

Mastoidectomy and Posterior Fossa Dural Exposure

A complete mastoidectomy is performed, skeletonizing the sigmoid sinus from the transverse sinus region inferiorly to the jugular bulb. The middle and posterior fossa dural plates are decompressed, and the facial nerve and semicircular canals are delineated. The facial nerve is left bony covered. In the retrolabyrinthine approach, decompression of the jugular bulb is performed, along with removal of the retrofacial/infralabyrinthine, retrolabyrinthine, and supralabyrinthine air cell tracts, resulting in complete skeletonization of the otic capsule bone. Exposure of the middle fossa dura facilitates removal of the middle fossa bone plate, and dural exposure along the middle fossa should extend from the root of the zygoma to the transverse-sigmoid junction. Full exposure of the superior petrosal sinus is critical, and all bony remnants should be carefully removed from this region as it is exposed from lateral to medial (**Fig. 8.3**).

Middle Fossa Craniotomy

Completion of the transmastoid drilling is facilitated by removal of the middle fossa bone plate. If dura can be easily stripped from the squamosa of the temporal bone, this can be accomplished using a craniotome. If there is any difficulty stripping, the

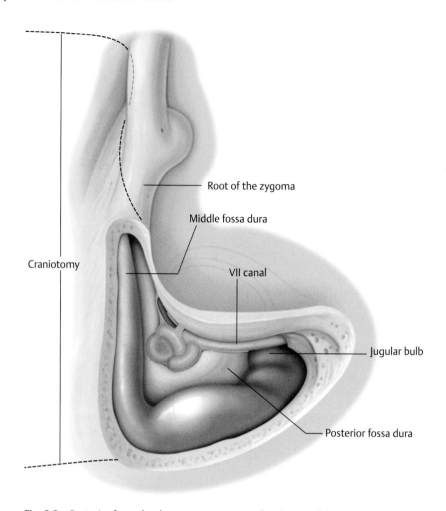

Fig. 8.3   Posterior fossa dural exposure, presigmoid in the retrolabyrinthine approach.

craniotomy can more safely be performed using a cutting bur. The bone flap is typically 5 × 6 cm, oriented vertically. It is made approximately four-fifths anterior to
the position of the external auditory canal position and one-fifth posterior to it. The
anterior limit of the craniotomy typically is the greater wing of the sphenoid bone.
A posterior/inferior extension of the craniotomy window may be performed to fully
decompress the middle fossa dura (**Fig. 8.4**). We do not typically perform a zygomatic
osteotomy, as anteroinferior retraction of the temporalis muscle over the zygomatic
arch region is usually sufficient to provide bony exposure of the root of the zygoma
and floor of the middle cranial fossa.

   After removal of the bone flap, the dura of the middle fossa floor is elevated from
posterior to anterior to protect the greater superficial petrosal nerve. The middle
meningeal artery is frequently coagulated and sectioned for access. The anterior limit
of the dural elevation is the dura over Meckel's cave and the medial limit of the dissection is the true petrous ridge and superior petrosal sinus.

   Once dural elevation is complete, a retractor is placed to retract the dura adjacent to
the superior petrosal sinus. This may be a House-Urban middle fossa retractor or a
Fukushima retractor. Drilling of the middle fossa floor is then performed. The superior
semicircular canal is skeletonized, as is the IAC. The bone of the petrous apex (Kawase's triangle) is removed, extending to the dura over Meckel's cave anteromedially
and to the carotid artery anterolaterally (**Fig. 8.5**). Air cells between the IAC and the
superior semicircular canal are exenterated, and the dura medial to this region is

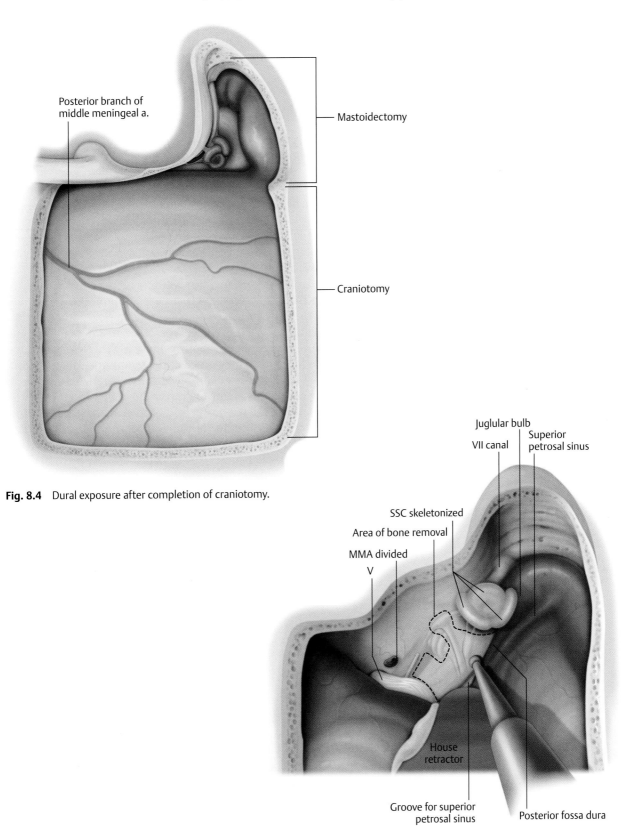

Fig. 8.4 Dural exposure after completion of craniotomy.

Posterior branch of middle meningeal a.

Mastoidectomy

Craniotomy

Juglular bulb

VII canal

Superior petrosal sinus

SSC skeletonized

Area of bone removal

MMA divided

V

House retractor

Groove for superior petrosal sinus

Posterior fossa dura

Fig. 8.5 Area of bone removal for the anterior petrosal or extended middle cranial fossa dissection. Bone removal can extend beneath the trigeminal nerve toward the petrous apex. MMA, middle meningeal artery; SSC, semicircular canal.

decompressed. The IAC dura is skeletonized laterally to the fundus of the IAC, taking care to prevent injury to the cochlea and the vestibule. The labyrinthine segment of the facial nerve is identified. Further details on the extended middle fossa exposure are described in Chapter 3.

Dural Incisions and Tumor Dissection

The first intradural exposure is made in the posterior fossa. A dural opening is carried out just anterior to the sigmoid sinus (**Fig. 8.6A**), and, if it is exposed, toward the IAC. The cerebellum is protected with a cottonoid as tumor is identified. It is critical to release cerebrospinal fluid (CSF) to relax the brain. Often, CSF flow is spontaneous. In other cases, it is necessary to dissect inferiorly to open the arachnoid layer of the cistern. It may also be necessary to resect a portion of the tumor at this time. Opening of the middle fossa dura should not be attempted until CSF is released from the posterior fossa and the brain is adequately relaxed. Generally, we also advocate identifying the facial and vestibulocochlear nerves at this stage.

Following adequate brain relaxation, the middle fossa dura is opened 1 cm lateral to the superior petrosal sinus (**Fig. 8.6B**). Cottonoids are used to protect the temporal lobe as retractors are used to gently elevate. With only minimal elevation, the tentorium can be followed to the incisura (**Fig. 8.7**). The trochlear nerve is identified, and the positions of any large arteries are noted. Bipolar cautery is used to coagulate the superior petrosal sinus, and the sinus is then divided. The tentorium is then divided, working laterally to medially. It is necessary to proceed slowly, cauterizing the dura in a stepwise fashion until the edge of the tentorium is reached at a location where the trochlear nerve can be seen. When the tentorium is fully opened, the cut edges usually separate, thus enhancing exposure into the superior portion of the posterior fossa. Care should be taken during opening of the tentorium to avoid injury to the trigeminal nerve, which may be pushed upward by tumor, and to any petrosal veins, which can be prophylactically coagulated.

With the tentorium opened, there is wide exposure of the superior portion of the posterior fossa, the region of the incisura, and the midbrain (**Fig. 8.8**). We utilize self-retaining retractors to gently elevate the temporal lobe when necessary. Retractors

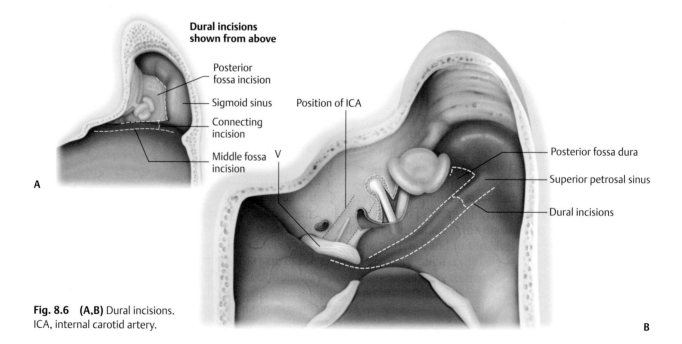

Dural incisions shown from above

Posterior fossa incision

Sigmoid sinus

Connecting incision

Middle fossa incision

Position of ICA

Posterior fossa dura

Superior petrosal sinus

Dural incisions

A

B

Fig. 8.6 (A,B) Dural incisions. ICA, internal carotid artery.

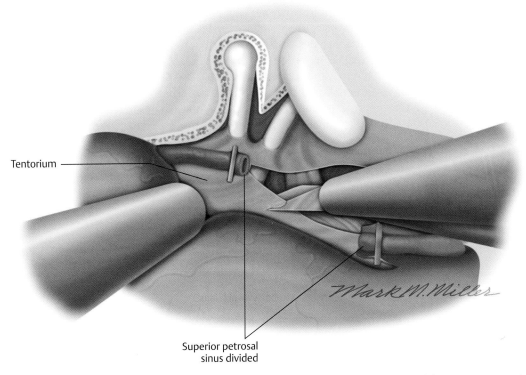

Fig. 8.7 The superior petrosal sinus is clipped and divided. The lateral to medial incision of the tentorium is made to the notch. Care must be taken to incise posteriorly within the notch to protect the trochlear nerve as it enters the tentorium anteriorly. Additionally, the surgeon must consider the vein of Labbé, as in some instances it travels with the leaves of the tentorium.

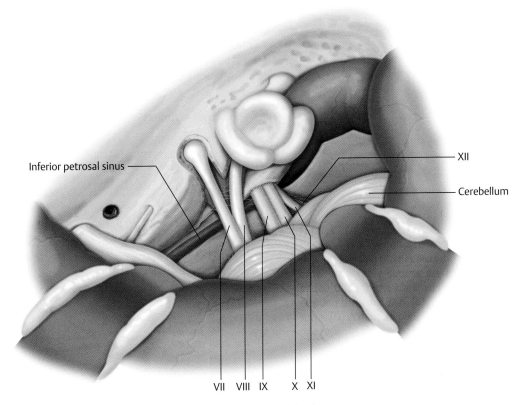

Fig. 8.8 Exposure of the posterior fossa after completion of dural incisions.

are not, however, used against the sigmoid sinus, which may be prone to thrombosis at this stage. Exposure may be facilitated with the removal of a pyramid-shaped portion of dura at the petrous apex above the IAC and lateral to the trigeminal nerve. This portion of dura includes the superior petrosal sinus, and care must be taken. However, with petroclival meningiomas, this portion of the sinus may already be occluded.

Tumor removal is undertaken with care. Central debulking is critical to dissect larger tumors from any cranial nerves or other important neurovascular structures. Dissection of the dural base of the tumor also helps to devascularize the tumor. However, blind coagulation of the dural base may be difficult with regard to several cranial nerves, notably the abducens, the course of which may not be fully appreciable until a significant portion of the tumor has been removed. This approach also provides excellent access to Meckel's cave, and tumor often can be safely removed from this region as well. We rarely if ever, however, make any attempt to remove tumor from the cavernous sinus.

Closure

After resection of tumor and the establishment of hemostasis, closure is performed. No attempt is made to close dura primarily. An onlay collagenous material may be used to reconstruct the middle fossa dura.

Once the tumor has been removed, abdominal fat is harvested from a left lower quadrant abdominal incision. A piece of dural replacement matrix is used to cover the area of resected dura along the inferior temporal lobe. Abdominal fat is used to pack the mastoid defect, as well as the cerebellopontine angle up to the region of the clivus. A piece of temporalis fascia is used to cover the mastoid antrum, in cases of hearing preservation, to prevent cerebrospinal fluid leak through the eustachian tube. In cases where the labyrinth has been sacrificed, the eustachian tube is obliterated with pieces of Surgicel Nu-Knit mixed with bone wax, and the middle ear is packed with muscle.

The temporal craniotomy bone flap is replaced, and plated into position with titanium miniplates and self-tapping screws. A piece of 1-mm titanium mesh is placed over the mastoid defect as a cranioplasty, and secured in place with screws. The musculopericranium is closed over the cranium, and the skin is closed in layers.

A loading dose of phenytoin is commonly given during the procedure, and maintenance doses are given intravenously or orally three times daily for 1 week postoperatively.

Variations

As mentioned previously, the posterior surgical approach may be extended as a partial labyrinthectomy (transcrusal), translabyrinthine, transotic, or transcochlear approach to improve surgical access to large tumors of the petroclival region. Tumors that extend significantly inferiorly along the clivus may require the additional exposure that resection of the labyrinthine bone provides.

Anatomic studies have shown that successive removal of labyrinthine bone beyond the retrolabyrinthine approach can provide more working room along the skull base to access more extensive tumors. Additionally, skeletonization of the carotid artery, jugular bulb, and jugular foramen is possible for tumors that extend to these areas.

Operative Pearls

Preservation of the Vein of Labbé

The drainage pattern of the vein of Labbé may be variable, but typically drains into the transverse sinus prior to the junction of the superior petrosal, transverse, and

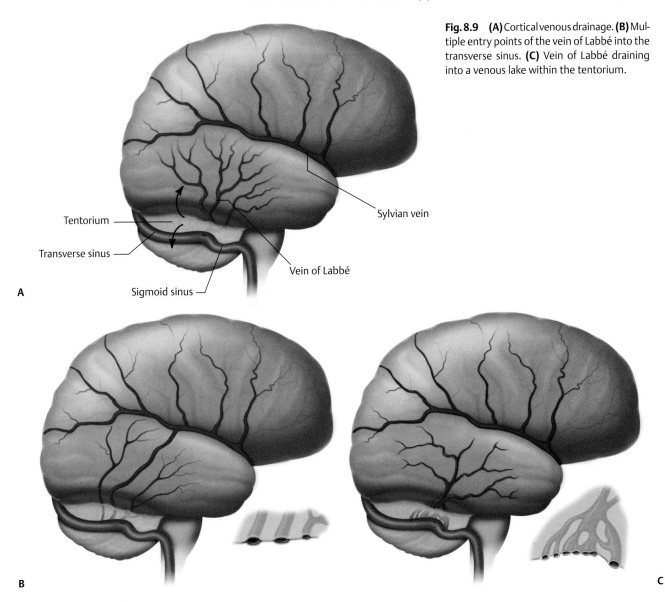

Fig. 8.9 **(A)** Cortical venous drainage. **(B)** Multiple entry points of the vein of Labbé into the transverse sinus. **(C)** Vein of Labbé draining into a venous lake within the tentorium.

Tentorium

Transverse sinus

Sigmoid sinus

Vein of Labbé

Sylvian vein

A

B

C

sigmoid sinuses. Variations on the venous anatomy have been reported from anatomic studies, and include the coalescence of draining veins into one vein (the venous candelabra), additional veins draining into the transverse sinus, or venous lakes in the tentorium served by the temporal draining veins (**Fig. 8.9**). Other variations may occur, with temporal bridging veins inserting into the superior petrosal sinus anterior to its junction with the transverse sinus. Transection of any draining veins or venous lakes is to be avoided. Depending on the anatomic variation, the petrosal approach may need to be modified or aborted.

Typically, the superior petrosal sinus is ligated or coagulated and divided anterior to its insertion into the transverse/sigmoid sinus junction, and the tentorium is cut in this location. The sigmoid sinus may also be divided; in this situation drainage of the vein of Labbé depends on the patency of the torcular and the contralateral transverse, sigmoid sinuses, and jugular veins and should be investigated with magnetic resonance venography (MRV) prior to surgery.

As temporal venous infarction can have devastating neurologic consequences, great care must be taken to preserve the venous drainage of the temporal lobe. Knowledge of its anatomic variations is essential to safe employment of the petrosal approach.

Table 8.2　Potential Complications of the Petrosal Approach

Cerebrospinal fluid fistula

Cerebrovascular accident

Seizure

Temporal venous congestion or infarction

Facial nerve palsy

Intracranial hematoma

Diplopia

Aphasia

Meningitis

Sensorineural hearing loss

Conductive hearing loss

Preservation of Cranial Nerve IV

Division of the tentorium cerebelli must be performed posterior to the insertion of cranial nerve IV into the dural folds. This must be balanced with the need to section the tentorium anterior enough to avoid any bridging veins that may enter the superior petrosal sinus or the anterior transverse sinus.

◆ Complications

As with all skull base procedures, the petrosal approach has potential complications that must be understood so that efforts may be made to prevent them, and when they do occur, that they may be recognized and dealt with effectively to minimize patient morbidity. Several potential complications are listed in **Table 8.2**.

◆ Conclusion

The combined petrosal approach is a versatile technique to approach lesions of the petroclival region. The variety of choices of an anterior and a posterior approach allow the surgical technique to be customized to the patient and to the lesion. Using bone removal of the lateral skull base allows for minimal brain retraction while increasing surgical exposure. The combined petrosal approach allows for removal of lesions of the petroclival region, particularly those with significant extension into the posterior cranial fossa.

Suggested Readings

Al-Mefty O, Fox JL, Smith RR. Petrosal approach for petroclival meningiomas. Neurosurgery 1988;22: 510–517

Cho CW, Al-Mefty O. Combined petrosal approach to petroclival meningiomas. Neurosurgery 2002;51: 708–716, discussion 716–718

Daspit C, Spetzler R, Detwiler P. Petrosal approach. In: Brackmann DE, ed. Otologic Surgery. Philadelphia: Saunders/Elsevier, 2010

Erkmen K, Pravdenkova S, Al-Mefty O. Surgical management of petroclival meningiomas: factors determining the choice of approach. Neurosurg Focus 2005;19:E7

Guppy KH, Origitano TC, Reichman OH, Segal S. Venous drainage of the inferolateral temporal lobe in relationship to transtemporal/transtentorial approaches to the cranial base. Neurosurgery 1997; 41:615–619, discussion 619–620

Horgan MA, Anderson GJ, Kellogg JX, et al. Classification and quantification of the petrosal approach to the petroclival region. J Neurosurg 2000;93:108–112

Sakata K, Al-Mefty O, Yamamoto I. Venous consideration in petrosal approach: microsurgical anatomy of the temporal bridging vein. Neurosurgery 2000;47:153–160, discussion 160–161

9

The Far Lateral Approach

Gregory P. Lekovic, Marc S. Schwartz, and Rick A. Friedman

The far lateral approach is less a single surgical approach than a family of approaches that can be tailored to individual pathology as needed. This versatility makes the far lateral approach, and its variations, the approach of choice for lesions of the inferior cranial base, extending from the internal auditory canal (IAC) superiorly to the cervicomedullary junction inferiorly and medially, and from the anterior lip of the foramen magnum to the jugular foramen and infratemporal fossa laterally. Because of the excellent exposure of the anterior foramen magnum and skull base provided by the approach, the far lateral approach can be employed in lieu of the more morbid transoral or transfacial approaches.

Common pathology treated via this surgical approach includes tumors of the cerebellopontine angle inferior to the IAC; glomus jugulare tumors, lower cranial nerve tumors, and other tumors of the jugular foramen; tumors of the inferior clivus; meningiomas of the foramen magnum; lateral and anterior intrinsic lesions of the medulla and upper cervical cord; and vascular lesions such as arteriovenous malformations and aneurysms of the vertebral arteries, posterior inferior cerebellar artery (PICA) origin, or vertebrobasilar junction.

Given this variety of pathology, it is perhaps not surprising that there is also a great deal of variation in the steps described in the literature as constituting elements of the far lateral approach. The first and most important concept in understanding this approach is that individualizing it is critical, and any particular maneuver, such as drilling of the occipital condyle or transposition of the vertebral artery, is not indicated in every case. For example, a large schwannoma of the jugular foramen may require less bony exposure than an aneurysm of the PICA, because in these cases the tumor has "done the dissection" for the surgeon.

◆ Classification of the Far Lateral Approach and Its Variations

The basic far lateral approach can be understood as simply an inferiorly and more laterally oriented retrosigmoid craniotomy. The occipital bone removed for the far lateral approach differs from a retrosigmoid craniotomy, however, in that the craniotomy extends to the foramen magnum. To this basic bone exposure, the following additional maneuvers may be added, depending on the individual case: (1) C1 hemilaminectomy, (2) drilling the occipital condyles, (3) transposition of the vertebral artery (or resection of the C1 transverse process), and (4) resection of the jugular tubercle and/or jugular process (**Table 9.1**).

Many variations of the far lateral approach have been described, encompassing many different maneuvers designed to increase exposure and obviate any retraction of eloquent structures. The far lateral approach is best understood by simplifying its classification into three categories: (1) the standard far lateral approach, in which a lateral suboccipital craniotomy is extended to the foramen magnum and a C1 hemilaminectomy is performed; (2) the transcondylar far lateral approach, in which the posterior occipital condyle is further drilled; and (3) the extended transcondylar ap-

Table 9.1 Classification of the Far Lateral Approach and Its Variations

Classification of Far Lateral Approach	Key Steps	Alternative Nomenclature	Paradigmatic Lesion(s)
Standard	Lateral suboccipital craniotomy with extension to foramen magnum; C1 hemilaminectomy	Retrocondylar (Sekhar); supracondylar (Rhoton); basic far lateral (Delashaw)	PICA aneurysm, glomus tumor, jugular foramen schwannoma
Transcondylar	Resection of posterior occipital condyle	Extreme lateral transcondylar (Sekhar); dorsolateral suboccipital transcondylar (Bertalanffy); transcondylar (Rhoton)	Foramen magnum meningioma, proximal PICA aneurysm
Extended transcondylar	Complete resection of condyle; and/or resection of jugular tubercle; jugular process; C1 lateral mass (i.e., transposition of vertebral artery)	Complete transcondylar, transjugular (Sekhar); complete far lateral suboccipital transtubercular (Day); ELITE (Couldwell); paracondylar (Rhoton)	Extensive clival/cranial base tumors, very high and anterior aneurysms of the proximal PICA or vertebrobasilar junction (VBJ)

proach, in which in addition to the foregoing additional bone is drilled, including the rest of the condyle exposing the hypoglossal canal, the jugular tubercle, the jugular process, or the transverse process of C1 (i.e., vertebral artery transposition). This classification reflects common clinical practice in that (1) resection of the occipital condyle is not always necessary, and (2) drilling the posterior third of the occipital condyle is usually all that is necessary to provide adequate anterior exposure. The extended transcondylar approach, including drilling of the entire occipital condyle, jugular tubercle, transposition of the vertebral artery, etc. is seldom necessary.

◆ Surgical Anatomy

The sternocleidomastoid muscle attaches superficially to the mastoid process and runs anteriorly. The suboccipital muscles have three distinct layers and attach widely to the mastoid and occipital bone. Surgeons should be familiar with the anatomy of the occipital triangles; a standard anatomy textbook should be consulted for this purpose if necessary. In practice, though, this "layer-by-layer" anatomy is not seen, as the muscles of the suboccipital triangle are elevated together from their periosteal attachments.

If the skin incision is extended into the neck for infratemporal fossa dissection, care must be taken not to injure the spinal accessory nerve, which lies anterior to the belly of the sternocleidomastoid muscle and emerges superficially at its anterior border. Similarly, care must be taken in elevating the digastric muscle from its groove in the posterior mastoid. The very anterior aspect of the attachment of the digastric muscle is in close proximity to the stylomastoid foramen and the exiting facial nerve. The occipital artery and nerve run between the middle and deep suboccipital muscles. Generally, it is necessary to divide these to attain sufficient inferior exposure.

Continuing to the deeper structures, the V3 segment of the vertebral artery begins as the artery leaves the foramen transversarium at C1 and enters the sulcus arterio-

Table 9.2   Surgical Landmarks

Bone	Muscle	Nerve	Artery	Vein
Asterion, occipito-mastoid suture	SCM/trapezius	Occipital nerve, accessory nerve	Occipital artery	
Digastric groove, mastoid tip	Digastric	Facial nerve at stylomastoid foramen		
Sulcus arteriosus of C1 lamina	Muscles of occipital triangle	C2 ganglion and dorsal ramus	V3 segment of vertebral artery	
C1 transverse process				Jugular vein
Occipital condyle, hypoglossal canal		Hypoglossal nerve		Condylar vein
Jugular tubercle and process				Jugular bulb

sus of the posterior arch of C1. Typically, the vertebral artery pierces the dura laterally, in line with the medial border of the lateral mass of C1; however, significant anatomic variation exists. Careful consideration of preoperative imaging is critical to minimize injury to the vertebral artery by allowing for preoperative identification of anomalous courses of the artery. Common variations in the anatomic relationships of the vertebral artery include circumferential ossification of the sulcus arteriosus (so that the artery traverses a bony canal) and an ectatic course of the artery, in which the sulcus is underdeveloped, or even absent, and the artery is freely mobile in the occipitocervical space. Although the vertebral artery gives off muscle branches in the neck, the surgeon must also be aware that in a minority of cases the PICA origin may be extradural. The V4 segment of the vertebral artery pierces the dura posteromedially and runs anteriorly around the brainstem before turning its course superiorly. All of the cranial nerves are superficial to the course of the vertebral artery.

The jugular process of the occipital bone forms the floor of the jugular foramen; that is, it is located posterior and inferior to the jugular foramen. The occipital condyle and the occipitocervical joint lie just below. The hypoglossal canal is located at the junction of the posterior and middle thirds of the occipital condyle and is oriented laterally approximately 45 degrees oblique to the sagittal plane. The intracranial foramen of the hypoglossal canal is located approximately 8 mm anterior to the posterior edge of the condyle. The most important surgical relationship of the jugular tubercle is that it is located between the hypoglossal canal and the jugular bulb.

Important intradural structures other than the vertebral artery include the lower cranial nerves. The hypoglossal nerve often crosses the vertebral artery at the origin of the posterior inferior cerebellar artery. The accessory nerve joins the vagus nerve, and these two nerves exit the dura together and run posteromedially through the jugular foramen. The glossopharyngeal nerve is usually separated from these two by a dural septum and runs anteromedially through the foramen (**Table 9.2**).

◆ Preoperative Workup

For resection of lesions of the jugular foramen, we routinely inspect the vocal cords preoperatively via direct laryngoscopy to identify preoperative vocal cord paresis. Patients may present with paresis or even paralysis of a vocal cord without significant hoarseness, particularly if the paresis has developed incrementally and the patient has fully compensated for the weakness. In this case, the risk of symptomatic lower cranial neuropathy is significantly reduced, and radical resection of jugular foramen lesions may be entertained.

When contemplating resecting the C1 lamina, the occipital condyle, or in extended transcondylar approaches, a computed tomography angiogram (CTA) of the neck must be obtained preoperatively. The vertebral artery may have an anomalous course, and hence be subject to a higher risk of iatrogenic injury. For vascular lesions such as aneurysms or arteriovenous malformations, a preoperative CTA may be obtained in conjunction with thin-slice imaging of the entire head to be used for image guidance. This may be particularly useful in partially embolized arteriovenous malformations (AVMs) where the embolisate can serve as a useful guide to feeding vessels. It is not necessary to obtain dynamic spinal imaging unless there is a specific reason to suspect preoperative spinal instability (e.g., erosion of the occipitoatlantal joint by tumor).

◆ Surgical Technique

Lumbar Drainage

Lumbar drainage is routinely employed both to ensure brain relaxation and to prevent postoperative pseudomeningocele formation and cerebrospinal fluid (CSF) leakage. Although it is classically taught that lumbar drainage may precipitate herniation if a block of free flow of CSF at the foramen magnum is suspected, in our experience lumbar drainage is safe as long as precautions are in place to ensure that not too much CSF is released prior to opening the dura. We typically leave lumbar drains in place for several postoperative days to aid with wound healing and to prevent postoperative leakage.

Monitoring

Facial nerve monitoring is utilized for all patients undergoing far lateral craniotomy. Glossopharyngeal and vagus nerve monitoring are also performed routinely. Monitoring of the glossopharyngeal nerve is accomplished with an electrode pair carefully inserted in the soft palate, and vagus nerve monitoring, although not consistently reliable, is performed utilizing endotracheal tubes with embedded electrodes. Electrical stimulation of the spinal accessory nerve in the unparalyzed patient results in a palpable shoulder contraction. Electromyography (EMG) electrodes are unnecessary.

Auditory brainstem monitoring is used not only for patients in whom hearing-preservation surgery is performed, but also routinely as a general indicator of brainstem integrity, and is of particular value when dealing with intrinsic brainstem lesions. Spinal cord somatosensory evoked potential (SSEP) monitoring is helpful both to detect long-tract compromise as well as positioning complications, such as brachial plexopathy. Motor evoked potentials (MEPs) are sensitive indicators of brainstem and anterior spinal cord integrity and are required for intrinsic brainstem lesions. Baseline SSEP and MEP runs are obtained prior to positioning.

Anesthetic Considerations

Perioperative antibiotics (usually cefuroxime 1.5 g IV) are given at the start of surgery and continued for 24 hours. Dexamethasone 4 mg IV q6 hours is also administered. Compression stockings are placed prior to induction of general anesthesia. Due to the use of cranial nerve monitoring, muscle relaxants are avoided or eliminated. If MEP monitoring is utilized, total intravenous anesthesia may be necessary.

Positioning

The patient is placed in either the lateral position (i.e., modified park bench) or the supine position with the head turned; the latter position is generally reserved for less extensive variations of the approach. In general, the patient should be positioned with the following objectives in mind: (1) to maximize ease of access to the surgical corridor, (2) to facilitate illumination, (3) to promote brain relaxation, and (4) to maximize surgeon comfort. A key factor in determining the ease of access to the surgical corridor is to minimize the degree of obstruction by the ipsilateral shoulder.

For the modified park bench position, the patient is placed in rigid three-pin fixation with a Mayfield head holder while still supine. The patient is then slid up on the table and turned in the lateral decubitus position on an axillary roll and with the dependent arm padded and placed in a sling. A Plexiglas board is extended over the edge of the bed and a beanbag may be used as well, to provide additional support. The head is then rotated 45 degrees toward the contralateral shoulder, flexed such that the chin is near to touching the clavicle, and laterally flexed 30 degrees (vertex down) to increase as much as possible the angle between the mastoid and the ipsilateral shoulder. The sum product of these maneuvers is to bring the clivus perpendicular to the floor, and allow the surgeon to look down the long access of the brainstem and work between the lower cranial nerves.

Skin Incision

Multiple skin incisions for the far lateral approach have been described, including "hockey-stick," "lazy S," and simple paramedian linear incisions. The traditional hockey-stick skin incision extends from the C2 or C3 in the midline superiorly to the superior nuchal line, then curving anteriorly, laterally, and inferiorly to the mastoid tip. A straight paramedian incision may also be employed, extending roughly from a line bisecting the line between the asterion and the external occipital protuberance to just posterior to the transverse process of C1 (which can usually be palpated readily).

The advantages of the hockey-stick incision over the paramedian incision are (1) the dissection proceeds from medial to lateral, and hence the vertebral artery is approached more safely; and (2) should atlanto-occipital fixation be required, the same midline segment of the incision may be utilized. It is, however, more time-consuming and arguably more traumatic for the patient. The lazy-S style incision is less traumatic and still allows for medial to lateral dissection at C1, but is essentially limited to lesions that do not extend into the infratemporal fossa, such as when there is no need to extend the incision into the neck (**Fig. 9.1**).

Monopolar cautery is used to develop a plane below the superficial muscle fascia. A small muscle cuff is cut and left attached to the superior nuchal line for reapproximation of tissues at the end of the procedure. The midline dissection is carried down the avascular ligamentum nuchae, and the muscle flap is reflected inferolaterally.

Variations

Lateral Suboccipital Approach

Although many surgeons would not consider a purely lateral suboccipital approach to be a far lateral approach, we include its description here to emphasize that resection of the C1 lamina and/or extension of the suboccipital craniotomy to the foramen magnum are not necessary in every case where a lateral trajectory is desired.

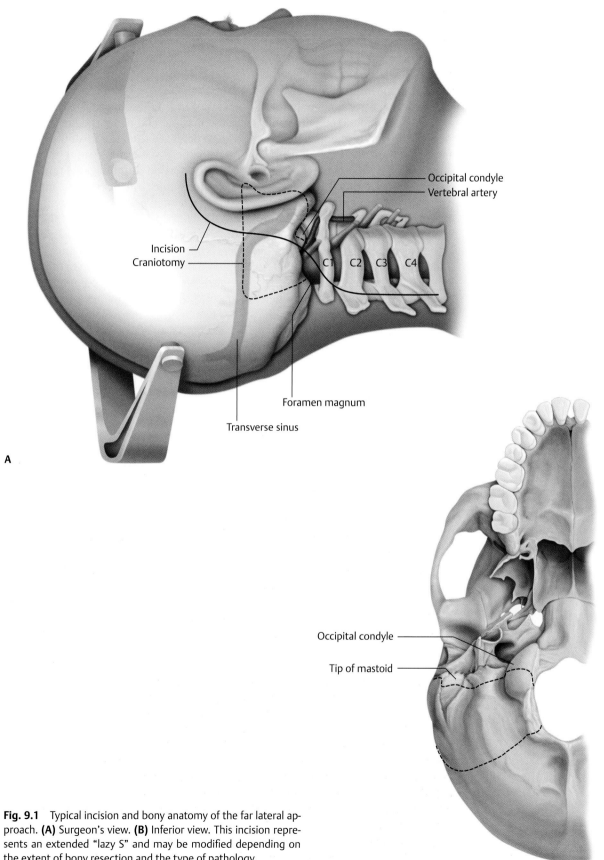

Fig. 9.1 Typical incision and bony anatomy of the far lateral approach. **(A)** Surgeon's view. **(B)** Inferior view. This incision represents an extended "lazy S" and may be modified depending on the extent of bony resection and the type of pathology.

For this variation, we typically position the patient supine with the head turned. A Mayfield headholder is used, and the head is rotated 45 to 60 degrees. The skin incision is similar to that made for a retrosigmoid craniotomy. However, the inferior limb of the incision may be extended along the anterior border of the sternocleidomastoid muscle, facilitating dissection into the neck along the courses of the lower cranial nerves and the internal jugular vein if necessary.

As with the retrosigmoid approach, the scalp flap is raised in the subgaleal plane toward the mastoid. The periosteum over the mastoid and along the nuchal line is incised. The sternocleidomastoid muscle can be detached from the tip of the mastoid and raised together with the scalp flap. The superficial suboccipital muscles are elevated medially and inferiorly. The most superior portion of the digastric muscle is elevated from its groove; however, dissection of this muscle is not carried anteriorly to the tip of the mastoid to avoid injury to the facial nerve. Inferior to the tip of the mastoid, the suboccipital muscles must next be divided along the course of the fibers. This is best accomplished using sharp dissection with Metzenbaum scissors. The fascia between the superficial and middle layers is opened, as is the bulk of muscle in the middle layer. The occipital artery is encountered in the plane just deep to the middle layer. This vessel must invariably be coagulated and divided. Dissection of the deep muscular layer is unnecessary when approaching the jugular foramen region.

For tumors that extend through the jugular foramen, into the temporal bone, or into the neck, mastoidectomy is performed. The retrofacial air cells are drilled out and the descending portion of the facial nerve is exposed. After carefully thinning the bone along the digastric ridge to the stylomastoid foramen, the tip of the mastoid can be removed (**Fig. 9.2**). This exposure can be further augmented by anterior translocation of the facial nerve, as discussed in Chapter 10. Exposure can also be augmented by labyrinthectomy or even more extensive transtemporal bone removal, if indicated.

Following mastoidectomy, the sigmoid sinus may be exposed to the transverse-sigmoid junction. This facilitates the performance of a retrosigmoid craniotomy based on the sigmoid sinus and the inferior aspect of the transverse sinus. The lateral suboccipital craniotomy is carried farther inferior than the standard retrosigmoid craniotomy, with the flap extending as far inferiorly as is comfortable. Additional bone is then removed to carry the bony opening to the horizontal portion of the occipital bone. In addition, bone may be removed using a diamond bur far enough to visualize the posterior border of the sigmoid sinus all the way to its curve anterior toward the jugular foramen (**Fig. 9.3**).

Exposure of the intracranial portion of tumor is gained via a suboccipital dural incision. The anterior dural flap, along with the unroofed sigmoid sinus, is retracted anteriorly using stay sutures. This provides additional exposure. Drainage of CSF to obtain brain relaxation is critical. As stated above, this can be ensured for larger tumors by using a lumbar spinal drain. Otherwise, elevation of the head may be helpful as the cerebellum is gently retracted using a small suction over a cottonoid. Because of the additional inferior exposure granted by the far lateral approach to the jugular foramen, this step is often easier than with the routine retrosigmoid approach. Arachnoid dissection is performed to separate the tumor from cerebellum. Care is taken to identify any lower cranial nerve fibers, which may be displaced posteriorly. The complex of cranial nerves VII and VIII is also usually displaced superiorly and posteriorly by tumors in this region. The vertebral artery is displaced anteriorly.

For jugular foramen tumors that have extensive extracranial involvement, the far lateral approach can be paired with a type A infratemporal approach. This is especially useful for schwannomas that grow along the lower cranial nerves. These tumors can often be totally resected. The most difficult portion of the tumor to fully visualize is the portion located in the jugular foramen proper. However, these tumors may enlarge the foramen, and by alternately viewing the foramen from both directions, tumor can be carefully mobilized and removed. Meningiomas extending extracranially

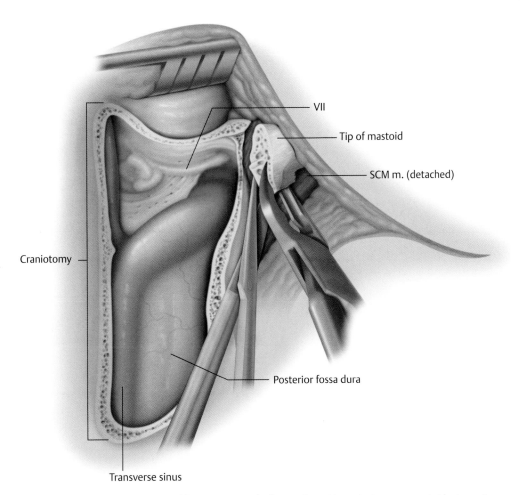

Fig. 9.2   Initial craniectomy. In addition to a standard retrosigmoid craniectomy, a mastoidectomy is performed, with particular attention to the inferior exposure. After identification of the facial nerve and digastric ridge, the mastoid tip is removed. SCM, sternocleidomastoid.

often extensively invade the surrounding structures. Total resection of these tumors is often impossible. Decompression of critical intracranial structures, rather than total tumor resection, may be the most appropriate goal for these tumors.

Standard Far Lateral Approach

In the standard far lateral approach the lateral suboccipital craniotomy is extended inferiorly to the foramen magnum and a C1 hemilaminectomy is performed. Removal of C1 in particular facilitates the inferior exposure by allowing the dura to be opened at a point much lower than is possible with a standard lateral suboccipital approach. By not resecting the occipital condyle, however, the standard far lateral approach offers limited anterior exposure.

The superior portion of the approach is identical to that performed for the retrosigmoid craniotomy. Inferiorly, much more extensive dissection is crucial. The more superficial layers of suboccipital muscle are detached from the mastoid and elevated posteriorly. Inferior to the tip of the mastoid, these muscles must next be divided along the course of their fibers. This is best accomplished using sharp dissection with Metzenbaum scissors. The fascia between the superficial and middle layers is opened, as is the bulk of muscle in the middle layer. The occipital artery is encountered in the plane just deep to the middle layer and is divided. Exposure in this area includes

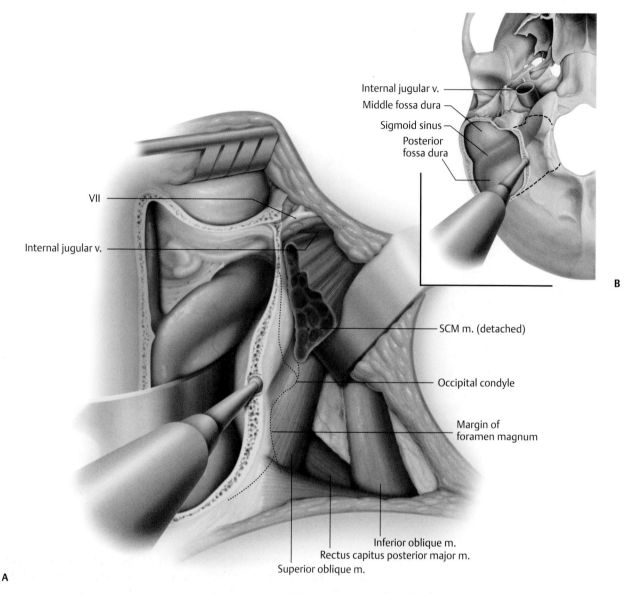

VII

Internal jugular v.

Internal jugular v.

Middle fossa dura

Sigmoid sinus

Posterior
fossa dura

B

SCM m. (detached)

Occipital condyle

Margin of
foramen magnum

Inferior oblique m.
Rectus capitus posterior major m.
Superior oblique m.

A

Fig. 9.3 Extension of inferior craniectomy. **(A)** The surgeon's view along the inferior sigmoid sinus beyond its anterior curve. **(B)** The extent of bony removal to the foramen magnum and posterior edge of the occipital condyle. SCM, sternocleidomastoid.

additional elevation of muscles from the suboccipital region. The occipital bone is widely exposed to the foramen magnum. Dissection is carried as far inferior as necessary to easily palpate the transverse process of C1 through the remaining deep layers.

The suboccipital muscles are elevated from their attachment at the lateral mass of C1. Care must be taken to avoid injury to the vertebral artery. This artery is surrounded by a plexus of veins, and venous oozing may be an issue. Some dissection of the vertebral artery along its course just above the arch of C1 to its entry into the dura is necessary, so understanding of its course is critical (**Fig. 9.4**). Subperiosteal soft tissue dissection is performed using elevators to expose the occipital bone and the arch of C1 all the way to the midline. With thinner patients, the inferior exposure in this region may be quite straightforward. With heavier patients, and especially those with well-developed musculature, this dissection may be much more difficult.

The authors typically start the bone dissection with the C1 hemilaminectomy. The posterior arch of C1 may be removed with a craniotome, rongeur, or diamond drill,

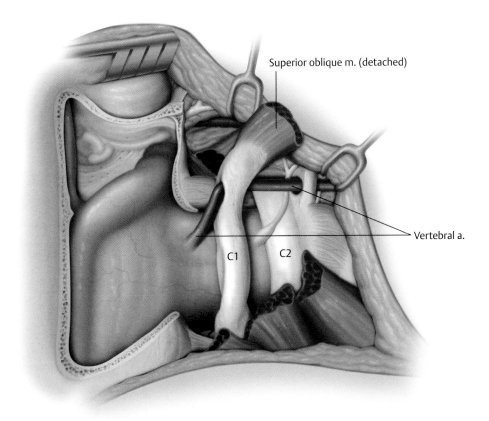

Superior oblique m. (detached)

Vertebral a.

C1   C2

Fig. 9.4 Exposure of the arch of C1. Muscle is detached at the lateral mass. The vertebral artery runs along the superior edge of C1 and is surrounded by a venous plexus.

depending on the surgeon's preference. The lateral aspect of the ipsilateral arch of C1 is then removed piecemeal, until the arch is felt and or seen to turn anteriorly, thus exposing the lateral border of the cervical dura (**Fig. 9.5**). The occipitoatlantal membrane is then dissected from the foramen magnum with a curved curette to allow for better definition of the inferior bony margin of the foramen magnum.

Next, the suboccipital bone is removed. Crossing the midline of the suboccipital bone may allow for ready access to the cisterna magna and for greater cerebellar decompression. We have found that a single bur hole placed on the keel of the suboccipital bone allows for efficient exposure of the dura; another bur hole can be placed right at the foramen magnum at the surgeon's option. Although we typically utilize cutting and diamond burs for bone removal, craniotomy may also be performed via bur holes and craniotome.

Once the bone work is completed, a semicircular dural incision is made, with the base of the semicircle reflected laterally, and held in place with stay sutures. The dural incision can be bisected if retraction is inadequate. The cerebellum is protected with a cottonoid as CSF is drained from the basal cistern. Direct exposure of the cistern facilitates CSF drainage and brain relaxation. Rather than performing extensive dissection of the extradural vertebral artery, this vessel is left within the surrounding soft tissue. Similarly, after opening the dura and draining CSF, epidural bleeding is often encountered; we therefore prefer not to open the arachnoid over the spinal cord until this has been controlled. Usually a hemostatic agent such as FloSeal (Baxter Healthcare Corp., Hayward, CA) and a cottonoid patty are sufficient. Once the arachnoid is opened, small hemoclips may be used to retract the arachnoid against the

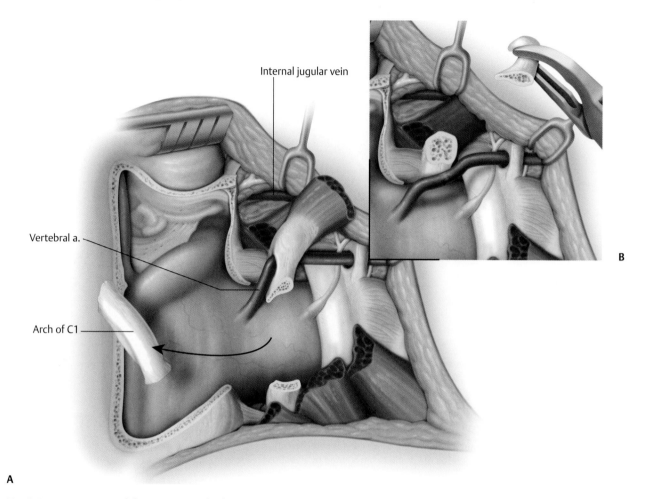

Internal jugular vein

Vertebral a.

Arch of C1

B

A

Fig. 9.5 Laminectomy of the posterior arch of C1. **(A)** Removal of medial bone. **(B)** Skeletonization of the vertebral artery. Degree of exposure at C1 and at the vertebral artery is tailored to the specific pathology and may not be necessary in all cases.

dura. The dentate ligaments are white fibrous bands that should be cut to allow for gentle retraction of the cervicomedullary junction. This also facilitates mobilization of the intradural vertebral artery.

The far lateral approach is most useful for lesions found anterior to the cranial nerves. This approach allows the surgeon to work between nerves without retracting or otherwise manipulating the brainstem and upper spinal cord. The paradigmatic lesion for this approach is meningiomas of the anterior foramen magnum (**Fig. 9.6**). Typically, the vertebral artery is displaced anteriorly by the tumor. The approach may allow early identification of this structure inferiorly, at its entry into the intradural space. Frequently, however, the artery is only identified after tumor resection begins (**Fig. 9.7**).

Transcondylar, Far Lateral Approach

The basic transcondylar, far lateral approach combines the standard far lateral approach described above with partial resection (i.e., the posterior one third to one half) of the occipital condyle. By removing the condyle, the surgeon is provided with an anterolateral trajectory to the brainstem. Without removing this bone, the dura cannot be retraced laterally sufficiently to expose the anterior brainstem. This approach thus provides access to lesions of the anterior foramen magnum, vertebrobasilar junc-

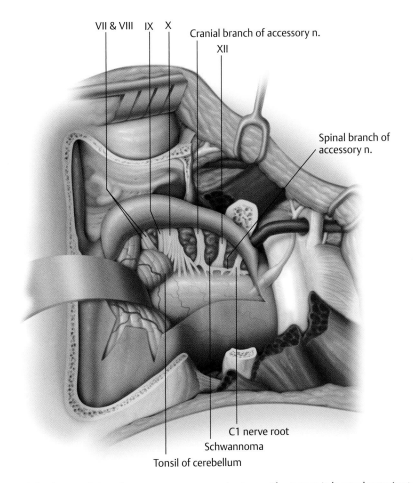

VII & VIII   IX   X   Cranial branch of accessory n.

XII

Spinal branch of
accessory n.

C1 nerve root

Schwannoma

Tonsil of cerebellum

Fig. 9.6 Approach to a foramen magnum meningioma. The tumor is located anterior to the cranial and spinal nerves. The lesion can be seen without retraction or manipulation of the brainstem or spinal cord.

tion, inferolateral pons, anterolateral medulla, and upper cervical spinal cord. Potential disadvantages of the transcondylar approach include vertebral artery injury, wound infection, meningitis, or lower cranial nerve deficits.

After performing the C1 laminectomy and suboccipital craniotomy as in the standard far lateral approach described earlier, the lateral foramen magnum is then drilled anteriorly until the posteromedial one third to one half of the occipital condyle is resected. This maneuver is most safely performed by drilling within the center of the condyle with a diamond bur under the microscope and leaving a thin eggshell of bone that can be removed with curettes or rongeurs. An excellent landmark for the extent of resection is the condylar emissary vein. The precise location of this vein in relationship to the condyle can usually be determined on preoperative thin-cut computed tomography (CT) studies. A good rule of thumb is that resection of the occipital condyle is inadequate until this vein is encountered. Although the vein can bleed prodigiously, it is easily controlled with bone wax. The hypoglossal canal, which should only be seen in the extended transcondylar exposure, is situated anterior and medial to the anterior third of the condyle.

Although resection of the posterior portion of the condyle usually does not result in occipitocervical instability, all patients should be evaluated with flexion/extension cervical x-rays. The presence of persistent neck pain postoperatively may be another sign of instability.

Vertebral a.

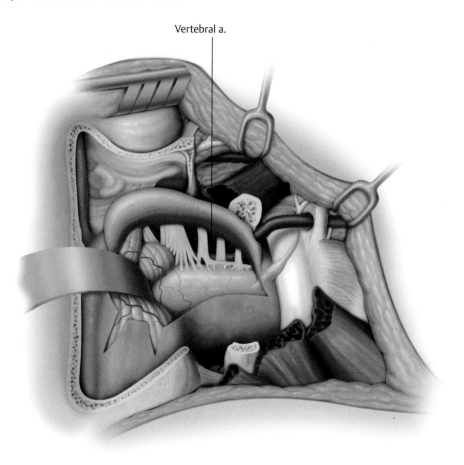

Fig. 9.7 View at the foramen magnum after resecting tumor. The vertebral artery runs anterior to the tumor and is identified during tumor resection.

Extended Transcondylar, Far Lateral Approaches

Various maneuvers can be employed to extend the exposure provided by the far lateral approach. These are considered together as the extended transcondylar approaches.

◆ Complete Resection of the Occipital Condyle

Extensive drilling of the occipital condyle provides enhanced anterior exposure of the foramen magnum, as well as the contents of the hypoglossal canal itself. For many types of pathology, however, resection of the condyle provides limited additional exposure and risks instability. With extensive or complete resection of the occipital condyle, occipitocervical fusion for craniocervical instability is a distinct likelihood.

◆ Resection of the Jugular Process and Jugular Tubercle

Resection of the jugular tubercle can be performed either intradurally (in the same manner as intradural resection of the anterior clinoid process) or extradurally. The indications for doing so are limited, with the most common being exposure of PICA origin aneurysm. Occasionally, the jugular tubercle may be exceptionally prominent and require drilling for even more lateral lesions.

The jugular process is the lateral extension of the occipital bone lying immediately superior to the transverse process of C1 and forming the floor of the jugular foramen. Resection of the jugular process is a lateral extension of the suboccipital craniotomy below the jugular bulb. This is most often required for exposure of intrinsic jugular foramen lesions. The surgeon must be mindful of the location of the internal jugular vein. Even though in the case of large jugular foramen tumors the jugular bulb may be compressed, the internal jugular vein may receive significant collateral venous drainage.

◆ **Vertebral Artery Transposition**

Although rarely necessary, transposition of the vertebral artery allows for a very anterior dural opening at C1-C2; this provides exposure of the anterior dura and medulla at these cervical levels.

To transpose the artery, the extradural vertebral artery, which lies on top of the sulcus arteriosus, is followed into the foramen transversarium with a Woodson or dental instrument. The foramen transversarium is then unroofed using either rongeurs or diamond burs. This mobilizes the vertebral artery so that it can be retracted medially and inferiorly. The lateral mass of C1 and the C1-C2 joint can then be inspected visually, allowing for resection of the C1 lateral mass. Sacrifice of the C2 nerve root is occasionally necessary. The venous plexus surrounding the vertebral artery can be the source of significant bleeding.

Closure

Closure of the far lateral craniotomy is performed carefully, with the prevention of CSF leak as the main goal. Primary closure without stretching of the dura or constriction of the intradural space is usually impossible. Instead, a primary closure with a suturable dural graft such as bovine pericardium or other suturable dural substitute is used. Alternatively, the dura may be loosely tacked together and reinforced with an onlay collagenous graft. Abdominal fat is used to fill all dead spaces, and the skull is reconstructed using the craniotomy flap and titanium mesh. The scalp is closed in overlapping layers, with particular attention to the lower portion of the incision, which is generally the most tenuous. Prophylactic lumbar drainage for several days promotes wound healing and may help prevent development of a pseudomeningocele.

◆ **Technical Pearls**

- The main goal of positioning is to remove the ipsilateral shoulder as a potentially source of hindrance to the surgeon.
- Inspect preoperative imaging to understand the anatomy of the vertebral artery and any possible anatomic variants.
- Tailor the extent of bone removal to the individual pathology, to ensure adequate but not overly aggressive dissection.
- Occipitocervical fusion is generally not necessary if less than half of the occipital condyle is resected; however, all patients undergoing any resection of the occipital condyle must be assessed postoperatively due to the possibility of instability.
- Lumbar spinal drainage is helpful not only to facilitate intraoperative exposure but also to promote wound healing and to prevent CSF leak.

◆ **Conclusion**

In properly selected cases and with sound preoperative assessment, the far lateral approach is a versatile approach to lesions of the lateral and anterior skull base. It is the approach of choice for vascular lesions of the proximal intracranial vertebral artery and vertebrobasilar junction, and is a powerful approach for tumors of the inferior-lateral skull base, such as jugular foramen tumors. Furthermore, the extreme lateral trajectory of the far lateral approach provided by the transcondylar and extended transcondylar variations makes it an attractive alternative to inferior anterior skull base lesions rather than more morbid anterior approaches, such as transoral or transfacial approaches.

Suggested Readings

Heros RC. Lateral suboccipital approach for vertebral and vertebrobasilar artery lesions. J Neurosurg 1986;64:559–562

Lanzino G, Paolini S, Spetzler RF. Far-lateral approach to the craniocervical junction. Neurosurgery 2005;57(4, Suppl)367–371, discussion 367–371

Sen CN, Sekhar LN. An extreme lateral approach to intradural lesions of the cervical spine and foramen magnum. Neurosurgery 1990;27:197–204

Spektor S, Anderson GJ, McMenomey SO, Horgan MA, Kellogg JX, Delashaw JB Jr. Quantitative description of the far-lateral transcondylar transtubercular approach to the foramen magnum and clivus. J Neurosurg 2000;92:824–831

Wu A, Zabramski JM, Jittapiromsak P, Wallace RC, Spetzler RF, Preul MC. Quantitative analysis of variants of the far-lateral approach: condylar fossa and transcondylar exposures. Neurosurgery 2010; 66:191–198

10

The Fisch Infratemporal Fossa Approach: Type A

William H. Slattery and J. Walter Kutz, Jr.

The infratemporal fossa type A approach allows safe access to the infralabyrinthine temporal bone, petrous apex, mandibular fossa, and posterior infratemporal fossa. It is a combination craniotemporal-cervical approach and requires anterior transposition of the facial nerve. This approach is used primarily for removal of glomus jugulare tumors; however, extensive cholesteatomas involving the internal auditory canal and petrous apex, lower cranial nerve neuromas, and carotid artery aneurysms may be approached in a similar manner.

Ugo Fisch initial proposed a classification system for categorization of these tumors (**Table 10.1**). This classification system is based on the extent of temporal bone involvement and intracranial extension of the tumor. Other classification systems have been proposed (**Tables 10.2 and 10.3**), but the Fisch system is still the most commonly used system.

Fisch first described the infratemporal approach to the infratemporal fossa and petrous apex in 1978. He subsequently reported the results of this technique in the management of 74 glomus jugulare tumors. The authors have made minor variations in the originally described technique. The basic steps are as follows:

1. Closure of the external auditory canal and removal of middle ear contents
2. Mastoidectomy with identification of the entire mastoid and tympanic segments of the facial nerve
3. Ligation of the jugular vein and identification of the internal carotid artery in the neck
4. Identification of the lower cranial nerves
5. Ligation or packing of the proximal sigmoid sinus
6. Transposition of the facial nerve from the geniculate ganglion to the parotid facial nerve
7. Removal of the tumor
8. Meticulous closure of the defect to prevent cerebrospinal fluid (CSF) leak

With careful surgical planning, gross tumor removal is often attainable with minimal morbidity. Persistent mild facial nerve paresis may occur (House-Brackmann grade 2 to 3); however, grade 1 facial nerve function can be achieved after facial nerve transposition. The risk of lower cranial nerve dysfunction is correlated with the size of the tumor and may present with postoperative dysphasia, hoarseness, or aspiration. Carotid artery involvement should prompt preoperative investigation of cerebral blood flow using balloon occlusion angiography.

◆ Preoperative Workup

A thorough history and physical examination are essential. A history of flushing, palpitations, and hypertension may suggest a secreting paraganglioma. Approximately

Table 10.1　Fisch Classification of Glomus Tumors

Class A	Limited to promontory of middle ear
Class B	Involves hypotympanum and mastoid, but cortical bone over the jugular bulb is intact
Class C1	Tumor erodes carotid foramen, but does not involve the carotid artery
Class C2	Tumor involves the vertical petrous carotid artery between the carotid canal and the carotid bend
Class C3	Tumor extends along the horizontal petrous carotid artery but does not involve the foramen lacerum
Class C4	Tumors extends across the foramen lacerum and the cavernous sinus
Class De1	Displace posterior fossa dura <2 cm
Class De2	Displace posterior fossa dura ≥2 cm
Class Di1	Intradural extension <2 cm
Class Di2	Intradural extension ≥2 cm
Class Di3	Neurosurgically unresectable

1% of glomus jugulare tumors actively secrete catecholamines. We routinely perform a 24-hour collection of urine to test for vanillylmandelic acid, norepinephrines, or metanephrines. If the 24-hour urine test is positive, a workup for multiple paragangliomas is warranted because glomus jugulare tumors rarely secrete catecholamines. In addition, careful perioperative planning with secreting tumors is necessary to prevent potentially devastating complications during surgery from the sudden secretion of catecholamines.

Both computed tomography (CT) and magnetic resonance imaging (MRI) with gadolinium should be utilized to fully evaluate the lesion. Bony architecture can be best appreciated in detail with CT, and involvement of the fallopian canal, petrous carotid artery, and the caroticojugular spine can be accurately evaluated. MRI with gadolinium contrast can best define soft tissue involvement and any intracranial involvement. In addition, MRI is extremely helpful in determining the status of the carotid artery in relationship to the tumor as well as the involvement of the cavernous sinus, infratemporal fossa, and sigmoid sinus.

Cerebral angiography with embolization is recommended for all tumors greater than Fisch class C1. Embolization can decrease intraoperative blood loss considerably and entail less blood in the operative field. Balloon occlusion of the internal carotid artery should be considered if preoperative imaging demonstrated possible involvement of the carotid artery. A slight risk of cerebrovascular accident is associated with balloon occlusion and should be taken into account.

Table 10.2　De la Cruz Classification Scheme for Glomus Tumors

Anatomic Classification	Surgical Approach
Tympanic	Transcanal
Hypotympanic	Mastoid-extended facial recess
Jugular bulb	Mastoid-neck (fallopian bridge technique or partial facial nerve rerouting)
Carotid artery	Infratemporal fossa
Transdural	Infratemporal fossa/intradural

Table 10.3 Glasscock and Jackson Classification of Glomus Jugulare Tumors

Type I	Small tumor involving the jugular bulb, middle ear, and mastoid
Type II	Tumor extending under the internal auditory canal; may have intracranial extension
Type III	Tumor extending into petrous apex; may have intracranial extension
Type IV	Tumor extending beyond the petrous apex into the clivus or infratemporal fossa; may have intracranial extension

Approximately 10% of patients present with multiple tumors. If multiple tumors are suspected, a whole-body octreotide scan is a useful screening tool. Although exceedingly rare, metastasis will be appreciated with an octreotide scan.

Preoperative antibiotics are administered and continued for 24 hours. Facial nerve and lower cranial nerve monitoring is performed on all cases. Glossopharyngeal electromyography (EMG) monitoring electrodes are placed. Long-acting muscle relaxants are avoided to prevent interference with cranial nerve monitoring. A lumbar drain may be placed in tumors with intracranial extension to decrease the incidence of postoperative CSF leak. The patient should be typed and screened for at least 4 units of blood. Autologous blood and the use of a cell-saver can reduce the amount of donor blood used.

◆ Surgical Anatomy

A thorough knowledge of temporal bone, jugular foramen, and cervical anatomy are essential to safely perform an infratemporal craniotomy. The anatomy of the temporal bone may be distorted due to tumor involvement. For instance, the vertical facial nerve may be displaced more laterally than usual due to lateral tumor extension. The middle ear space is often filled with tumor and covers the typical landmarks. Adequate preoperative imaging and preoperative planning can prevent complications in these incidences.

The internal carotid artery is usually intimately involved with tumor, requiring a familiarity with the anatomy. The internal carotid artery is initially identified in the neck and can be differentiated from the external carotid artery due to the lack of cervical arterial branches. Superiorly, the genu of the petrous internal carotid artery is medial and superior to the orifice of the eustachian tube. The caroticotympanic branch originates from the ascending petrous internal carotid artery and should not be avulsed during dissection.

The lower cranial nerves exit through the pars nervosa of the jugular foramen. The medial jugular bulb is preserved to create a safe plane between the lower cranial nerves and the tumor. The lower cranial nerves may be injured with overzealous packing of the inferior petrosal sinus opening into the medial wall of the jugular bulb. When packing or ligating the sigmoid sinus, the vein of Labbé should not be occluded. This can be prevented by packing the sinus distal to the superior petrosal sinus.

◆ Surgical Technique

The patient is placed in the supine position with the head turned away from the operative site. Facial nerve and glossopharyngeal EMG electrodes are placed for intraoperative monitoring. A C-shaped incision is performed two fingerbreadths from the postauricular sulcus, down to the mastoid tip, and continuing into the neck two fingerbreadths below the angle of the mandible (**Fig. 10.1**). An incision is then made

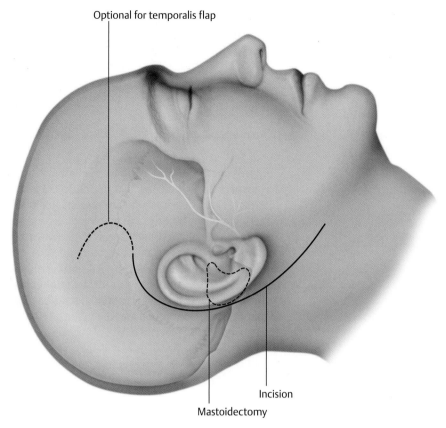

Optional for temporalis flap

Incision

Mastoidectomy

Fig. 10.1   The incision is made 4 cm postauricular. The apex of the incision is at the mastoid tip. The incision extends into the neck, two fingerbreadths below the mandible. An optional superior extension can be done if a temporalis flap is needed.

through the periosteum posterior along the linea temporalis and then inferior to the mastoid tip. The periosteum is elevated anteriorly and the external auditory canal is transected just medial to the bony-cartilaginous junction. The skin of the external auditory canal is then elevated away from the underlying cartilage. The skin of the canal is then everted and closed with interrupted 4–0 nylon sutures. The anterior-based periosteal flap is then closed over the canal to provide an extra layer of closure (**Fig. 10.2**). This results in a blind sac closure of the external auditory canal. The skin of the canal, tympanic membrane, malleus, and incus are now removed after the in-cudostapedial joint has been disarticulated.

A wide mastoidectomy is performed. The middle fossa dura, posterior fossa dura, and sigmoid sinus are identified. Caution must be taken while drilling medially be-cause the facial nerve may be displaced more laterally in a larger tumor involving the infralabyrinthine temporal bone. The facial nerve is skeletonized from the geniculate ganglion to the stylomastoid foramen (**Fig. 10.3**). The posterior external auditory ca-nal wall is removed, and the remaining tympanic ring is removed to allow adequate visualization of the jugular bulb, carotid artery, and the temporomandibular joint. All cancellous bone in the infralabyrinthine compartment is removed to prevent leaving small remnants of tumor in the bone.

The incision is then carried into the neck. The anterior border of the sternocleido-mastoid (SCM) muscle is identified. The mastoid tip is removed and the jugular vein, carotid artery, and cranial nerves IX, X, XI, and XII are identified. Ligatures are placed around the internal carotid artery and the internal jugular vein for identification and vascular control (**Fig. 10.4**). The facial nerve is identified as it exits the stylomastoid

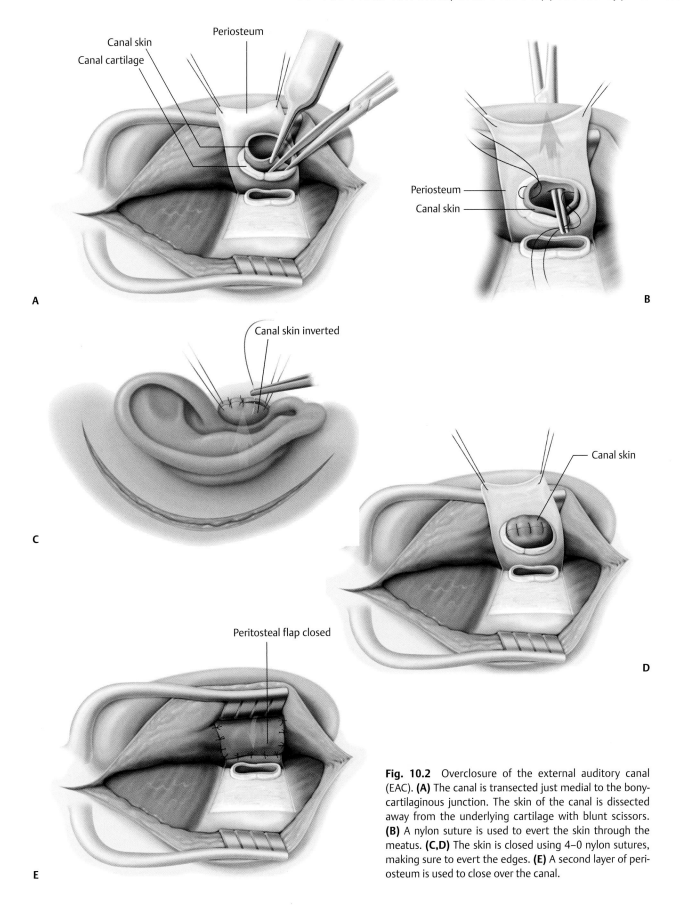

Fig. 10.2 Overclosure of the external auditory canal (EAC). **(A)** The canal is transected just medial to the bony-cartilaginous junction. The skin of the canal is dissected away from the underlying cartilage with blunt scissors. **(B)** A nylon suture is used to evert the skin through the meatus. **(C,D)** The skin is closed using 4–0 nylon sutures, making sure to evert the edges. **(E)** A second layer of periosteum is used to close over the canal.

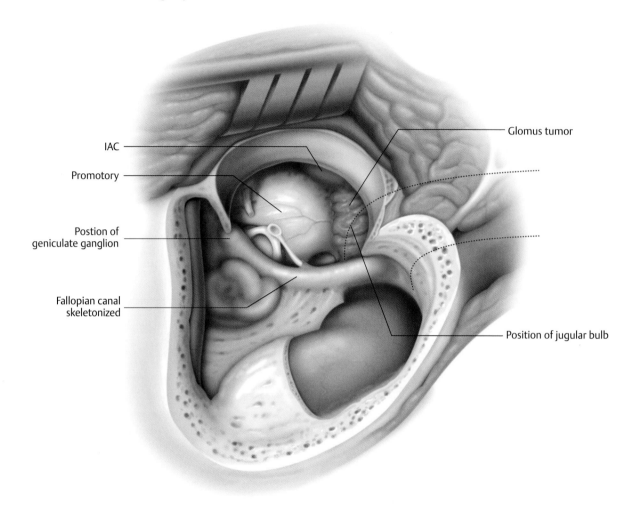

IAC

Promotory

Postion of
geniculate ganglion

Fallopian canal
skeletonized

Glomus tumor

Position of jugular bulb

Fig. 10.3 The skeletonized facial nerve with the lateral canal, sigmoid sinus, and posterior and middle fossa are shown. This drawing should be rotated counterclockwise 90 degrees to correspond to the surgeon's view. Also shown is a mastoidectomy with the posterior fossa dura and sigmoid sinus skeletonized. The sigmoid sinus should have a bone over it approximately 1 cm to the sinodural angle (where the middle fossa tegmen and sinus join). The posterior external auditory canal should be removed. IAC, internal auditory canal.

foramen. The posterior belly of the digastric muscle is then freed from the mastoid tip.

Next, the facial nerve is transposed from the geniculate ganglion to the stylomastoid foramen. The facial nerve has previously been identified and skeletonized. Removal of bone over the second genu should only include the bone adjacent to the middle ear cavity to prevent an inadvertent fistula of the lateral semicircular canal. Removal of the stapes suprastructure may be required to allow adequate access. After the facial nerve has been skeletonized, a sickle knife, Rosen needle, or Fisch microraspatory can be used to remove the remaining bone; 270 degrees of bone should be removed around the facial nerve in the mastoid segment and 180 degrees of bone removed around the tympanic and second genu before the nerve is dissected out of the fallopian canal. The facial nerve is then gently lifted from the fallopian canal in the mastoid segment until the medial attachments are encountered. Sharp dissection of these attachments prevents injury to the nerve and allows elevation to continue toward the geniculate ganglion (**Fig. 10.5**).

The facial nerve is firmly adherent to the periosteum of the stylomastoid foramen. To prevent injury, the periosteum should be included with the transposed facial nerve. The posterior belly of the digastric can be used to lift the nerve anterior. Once

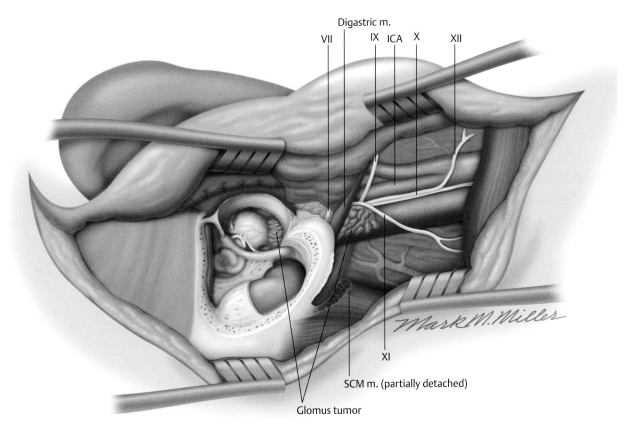

Fig. 10.4 Anatomy of the neck. The relationship of the jugular bulb, carotid artery, and cranial nerves IX through XII is demonstrated. The sternocleidomastoid (SCM) muscle has been retract posteriorly. Cranial nerve XI1 crosses over the jugular vein. Cranial nerve IX crosses over the carotid artery. ICA, internal carotid artery.

the facial nerve has been completely mobilized, it is placed anterior along the parotid gland, which has been freed from the attachments to the SCM. A small portion of parotid gland can be oversewn to hold the facial nerve in place. Tumor intimately involving the facial nerve should be removed with small scissors at the conclusion of the dissection. Removing the tumor when the nerve is not mobilized may result in stretch injury because the epineurium has been violated. The use of intraoperative facial nerve monitoring has greatly improved the results in procedures requiring facial nerve transposition.

The parotid gland attachments are then dissected away from the temporal bone. The final step to free the mandible is to remove the styloid process. Care must be taken not to injure the underlying carotid artery when fracturing the styloid process. Next a large Perkins retractor is placed from the angle of the mandible to the anterior border of the SCM. Care must be taken to prevent crushing the transposed facial nerve with the retractor. This maneuver exposes the infratemporal fossa and obviates the need to resect the mandibular condyle in most cases. The infralabyrinthine bone overlying the jugular bulb, carotid artery, and sigmoid sinus is removed.

The sigmoid sinus is next occluded proximally. If the tumor does not extend intradural, the bone overlying the sigmoid sinus distal to the insertion of the superior petrosal sinus is preserved. Oxidized cellulose is then packed firmly under the remaining bone to occlude the proximal sigmoid sinus. Care must be taken to prevent occlusion of the vein of Labbé, which could result in temporal lobe edema or an infarct. If the tumor is intradural, the sigmoid sinus is ligated. This is achieved by passing an aneurysm needle or hemostat under the sinus and ligating the sinus with a silk suture (**Fig. 10.6**).

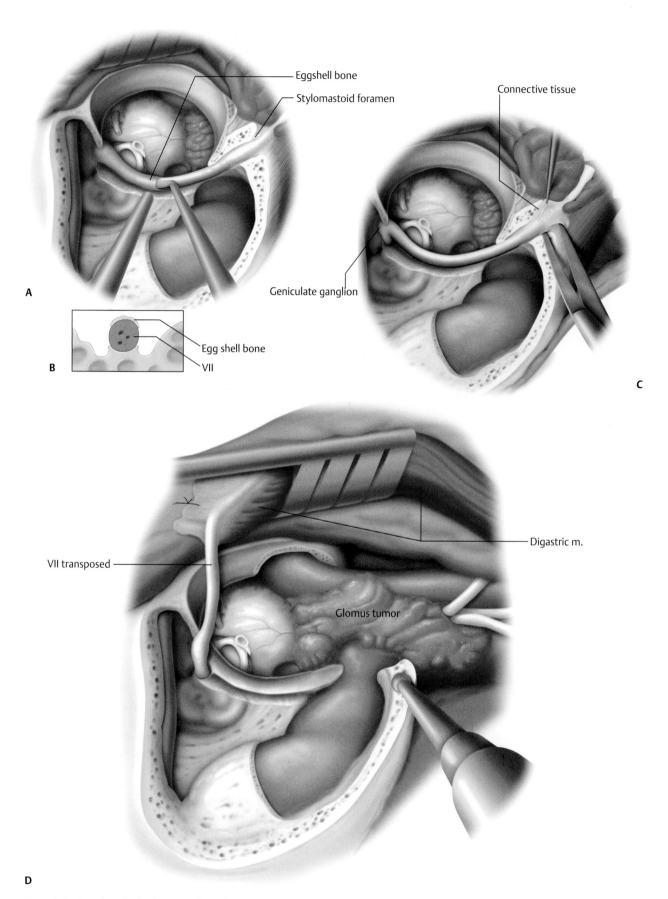

Fig. 10.5 **(A–D)** Multiple drawings show the removal of bone, medial attachments near the second genu and sharp dissection, the nerve transposed with the stylomastoid foramen periosteum, and the posterior digastric muscle.

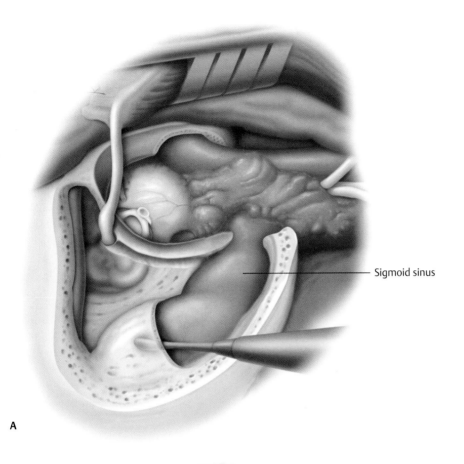

A

Sigmoid sinus

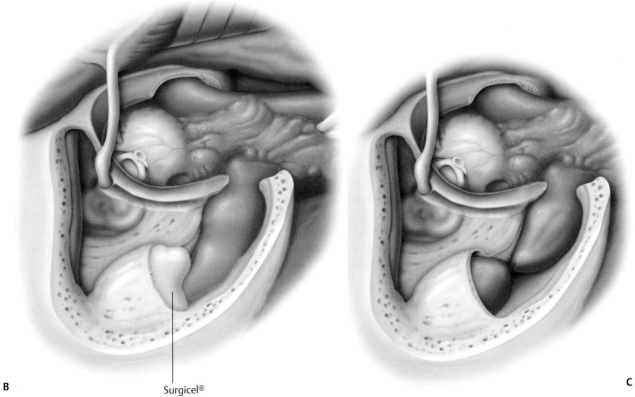

B

Surgicel®

C

Fig. 10.6   (A–C) Packing of the sigmoid sinus.

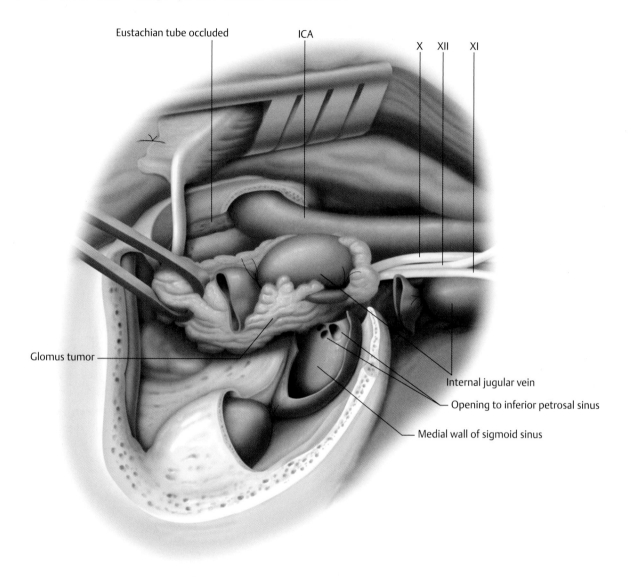

Eustachian tube occluded   ICA   X   XII   XI

Glomus tumor

Internal jugular vein

Opening to inferior petrosal sinus

Medial wall of sigmoid sinus

Fig. 10.7   Tumor involving the carotid artery. ICA, internal carotid artery.

The carotid artery distal to the tumor is identified. Next, the medial wall of the eustachian tube is removed to find the petrous carotid artery. Care must be taken not to injure a dehiscent carotid artery. The eustachian tube is then obliterated with muscle and/or bone wax. The carotid artery must be followed distal to the tumor to ensure safe removal of the tumor.

The jugular vein is now double ligated. The external carotid artery and branches distal to the lingual artery can also be ligated, including the ascending pharyngeal artery, which is a major blood supply of the tumor. The jugular vein is then passed under the spinal accessory nerve to the level of the jugular bulb. The tumor is then followed superior along the carotid artery with fine-tipped dissecting hemostats. The tumor often involves the periosteum of the carotid artery, which must be included with the specimen; however, adventitial involvement is uncommon. Tumor intimately involved with the carotid artery and the caroticotympanic branch should be dissected at the conclusion of the procedure to allow easier control of hemorrhage (**Fig. 10.7**).

The medial wall of the jugular bulb is a useful plane between the tumor and the lower cranial nerves. The inferior petrosal sinus empties into the jugular bulb in

Cellulose

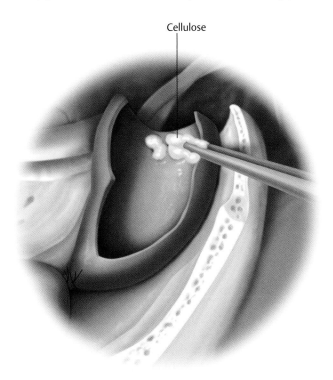

Fig. 10.8 The medial wall of the jugular bulb with multiple openings of the inferior petrosal sinus, and these opening are packed. Observe the close relationship of the lower cranial nerves.

multiple areas and can be controlled with oxidized cellulose packing (**Fig. 10.8**). The inferior petrosal sinus should be inspected before packing to prevent residual tumor. Also, overzealous packing can result in compression of the lower cranial nerves.

Intradural tumor is then removed if the patient is hemodynamically stable and has not lost an excessive amount of blood. A second-stage procedure is sometimes a better alternative. Once tumor removal has been achieved, the eustachian tube is pack with oxidized cellulose and a temporalis muscle plug. The dural defect is repaired and abdominal fat is used to obliterate the defect. A Penrose drain is placed and a pressure dressing is applied.

◆ Limitations

Limitations of the type A infratemporal approach are directed by anatomic and disease factors. Class A, class B, and select class C1 tumors may be treated with transcanal, transmastoid-extended facial recess, or mastoid-neck approaches. These approaches have the advantage of not transposing the facial nerve. Large tumors with intradural involvement are generally accessible through a type A approach. Tumors that involve the foramen lacerum or the cavernous sinus (class C4 tumors) are best approached with the type C infratemporal fossa approach (see Chapter 11). Carotid artery involvement that precludes removal of tumor without sacrifice of the artery should be avoided. Preoperative evaluation of large tumors should include balloon occlusion angiography to assess cerebral blood flow. Class Di3 tumors are defined as surgically unresectable due to extensive intracranial involvement or metastasis. Partial tumor removal followed by radiation therapy may be beneficial in select cases.

◆ Technical Pearls

- Preoperative evaluation should include angiography with embolization, and surgery should follow within 48 hours.
- Screening for secreting tumors will allow improved perioperative planning.
- Facial and glossopharyngeal nerve monitoring should be utilized.
- Autologous blood and the use of a cell-saver should be considered in any tumor large enough to be treated with a type A approach.
- The external auditory canal should be meticulously closed in two layers and done at the beginning of the procedure.
- Do not skeletonize the sigmoid sinus too proximally to prevent occluding the vein of Labbé when packing.
- When transposing the facial nerve out of the fallopian canal, use sharp dissection for the medial attachments.
- Tumor attached to the facial nerve should be removed at the end of the procedure because violation of the epineurium is more likely to allow stretch injury.
- Free the parotid gland attachments from the temporal bone and remove the styloid process to allow mobilization of the mandible.
- Do not inadvertently crush the transposed facial nerve with the retractor.
- Do not attempt to remove the facial nerve from the stylomastoid periosteum. Instead, keep the nerve attached to the periosteum and elevate anteriorly with the posterior belly of the digastric.
- Tumor often involves the periosteum of the carotid canal, but rarely invades the adventitia.
- Use the medial wall of the jugular bulb as a plane between the tumor and lower cranial nerves.
- The inferior petrosal sinus usually has multiple openings into the jugular bulb.
- Inspect the inferior petrosal sinuses for tumor before packing.
- Tumor involving the carotid artery and the caroticotympanic branch should be removed last. Troublesome bleeding can be handled with less difficulty.
- Meticulous closure should include closure of the dura and fat obliteration.

◆ Conclusion

The type A infratemporal fossa approach is utilized for lesions involving the jugular foramen, infratemporal fossa, and petrous carotid artery. This approach is a cranio-temporal-cervical approach affording wide access to the lateral skull base from the temporal bone to the upper neck. Thorough knowledge of the anatomy in this region is essential for successful removal of tumors and to prevent potentially catastrophic complications.

Suggested Readings
Brackmann DE. The facial nerve in the infratemporal approach. Otolaryngol Head Neck Surg 1987;97:
    15–17
Gadre AK, O'leary MJ, Zakhary R, Linthicum FH, House WF. The lateral skull base: a vascular perspec-
    tive with clinical implications. Skull Base Surg 1991;1:110–116
Green JD Jr, Brackmann DE, Nguyen CD, Arriaga MA, Telischi FF, De la Cruz A. Surgical management of
    previously untreated glomus jugulare tumors. Laryngoscope 1994;104(8 Pt 1):917–921
Horn KL, House WF, Hitselberger WE. Schwannomas of the jugular foramen. Laryngoscope 1985;95
    (7 Pt 1):761–765
Leonetti JP, Brackmann DE, Prass RL. Improved preservation of facial nerve function in the infratem-
    poral approach to the skull base. Otolaryngol Head Neck Surg 1989;101:74–78
Molony TB, Brackmann DE, Lo WW. Meningiomas of the jugular foramen. Otolaryngol Head Neck Surg
    1992;106:128–136

11

The Fisch Infratemporal Fossa Approach: Types B and C

Derald E. Brackmann and Robert D. Cullen

The infratemporal fossa is a well-guarded area of the skull base. The facial nerve and carotid artery are the main obstacles to accessing this region with minimal morbidity. Ugo Fisch developed a systematic approach to lesions of the infratemporal fossa in the 1970s. The type A approach, and modifications thereof, are utilized in accessing the jugular foramen and lesions medial to the facial nerve. As the type A approach is covered in Chapter 10, it will not be discussed further here. The type B approach allows access to the petrous apex, clivus, horizontal segment of the intratemporal carotid artery, and the posterior infratemporal fossa. Lesions anterior to the external auditory canal may be approached by leaving the facial nerve within the fallopian canal, thereby reducing the chance of paresis that may occur with the type A approach. The type C approach is an extension of the type B approach and allows access to the infratemporal fossa, pterygopalatine fossa, parasellar region, and the nasopharynx. The different exposures obtained with the Fisch types A, B, and C approaches are demonstrated in **Fig. 11.1**.

◆ Indications

Type B and C approaches provide exposure to benign lesions of the infratemporal fossa, petrous apex, and clivus. The decision to use these approaches in the treatment of malignancies involving the skull base should not be made lightly. Piecemeal removal of tumors should be expected. En bloc removal of tumors with adequate margins is usually not possible without producing significant morbidity. **Figures 11.1, 11.2, and 11.3** schematically demonstrate the anatomic exposure obtained in the type B and C approaches.

- Type B approach: benign lesions of the petrous apex, clivus, and posterior infratemporal fossa
- Type C approach: skull base lesions involving the infratemporal fossa, the pterygopalatine fossa, the parasellar region, and the nasopharynx

◆ Surgical Anatomy

The infratemporal fossa provides the most challenging anatomy for the skull base surgeon. Mastering the anatomy of the infratemporal fossa requires a thorough understanding of the bony, muscular, and neurovascular contributions to this area. The bony anatomy of the infratemporal fossa is demonstrated in **Figs. 11.4, 11.5, and 11.6**. Note the linear relationship of the mastoid tip, stylomastoid foramen, sphenoid spine,

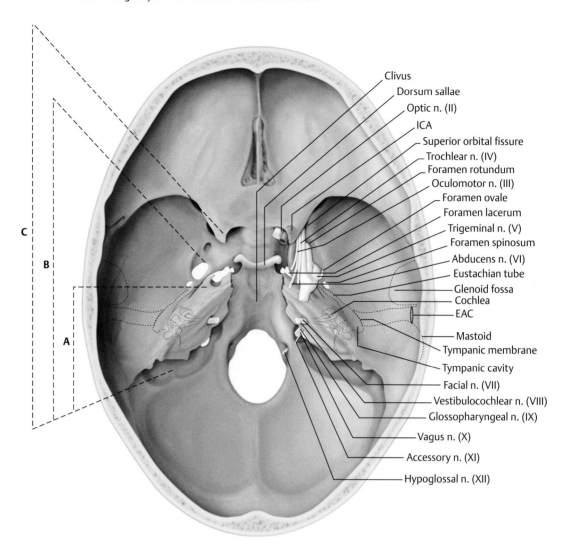

Fig. 11.1   The Fisch-described infratemporal fossa approach has three variations providing a graded level of anterior and medial exposure. The type A provides exposure to the region of the jugular foramen, the vertical segment of the internal carotid artery (ICA), and the posterior infratemporal fossa. The type B provides additional exposure to the petrous apex and horizontal ICA and the clivus. The type C provides an extension to the anterior infratemporal fossa, the nasopharynx, the pterygopalatine fossa, and the cavernous sinus. Pertinent skull base anatomy as seen above is labeled. EAC, external auditory canal.

foramen spinosum, foramen ovale, and the lateral pterygoid plate. The eustachian tube and carotid artery run parallel and medial to this line, with the carotid artery lying medial to the eustachian tube.

The muscles of the infratemporal fossa include the medial and lateral pterygoid muscles and the temporalis muscle. The temporalis muscle originates on the lateral surface of the skull, the temporal fossa, and the posterior border of the frontal process of the zygomatic bone. The blood supply originates from the maxillary artery via the deep temporal arteries. These arteries lie on the deep surface of the temporalis muscle and may be injured during elevation of the muscle if not carefully preserved. The lateral pterygoid muscle originates on the greater wing of the sphenoid and lateral aspect of the lateral pterygoid plate to insert on the medial mandibular neck. The medial pterygoid originates on the medial side of the lateral pterygoid plate and follows an inferior course as it inserts on the medial mandibular neck.

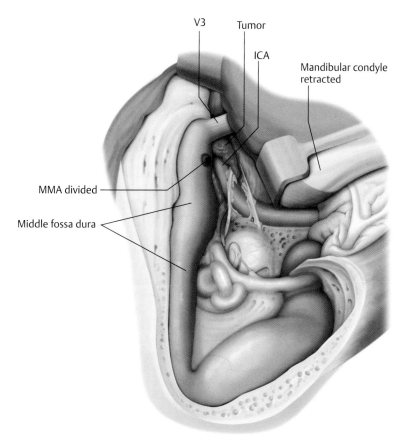

Fig. 11.2 Infratemporal fossa type B. The facial nerve is rerouted anteriorly, and the horizontal intrapetrous carotid artery is exposed to gain safe access to the petrous apex and clivus. This approach requires removal of the glenoid fossa, division of the middle meningeal artery (MMA), and division of V3. ICA, internal carotid artery.

The maxillary artery arises from the external carotid artery and passes medial to the ramus of the mandible (mandibular portion of the maxillary artery) to enter the infratemporal fossa (**Fig. 11.5**). It may course medial or lateral to the inferior head of the lateral pterygoid. This pterygoid portion of the maxillary artery give rise to the middle meningeal, inferior alveolar, pterygoid, masseteric, and deep temporal arteries. The maxillary artery then enters its pterygopalatine portion after passing through the sphenopalatine fissure. Great care should be taken to preserve the deep temporal arteries, as they provide the primary blood supply to the temporalis muscle.

An understanding of the fascial planes of the temporal region is also mandatory. There are three primary fascial layers within the temporal region that are of primary importance, particularly in their relationship to the facial nerve (**Figs. 11.7 and 11.8**). The temporoparietal fascia (superficial temporal fascia) is an extension of the superficial musculoaponeurotic system (SMAS) and is in continuity with the galea and frontalis muscle. This layer envelops the frontal branch of the facial nerve and the superficial temporal artery. The deep temporal fascia is composed of two layers: the superficial and deep layers. The superficial and deep layers of the deep temporal fascia split at the temporal line of fusion to envelop the zygomatic arch. The superficial temporal fat pad rests between these layers and extends down to the zygomatic arch. This fat pad provides an excellent landmark for the appropriate plane of dissection to access the zygoma and protect the frontal branch of the facial nerve.

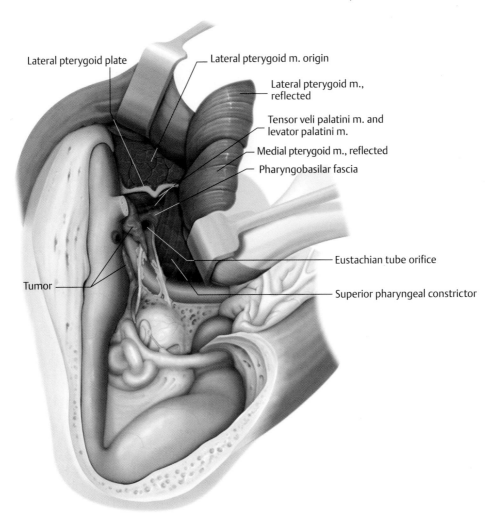

Fig. 11.3   Extension to the infratemporal type C approach. This allows access to the pterygopalatine fossa, the nasopharynx, and the cavernous sinus.

◆ **Surgical Technique**

Patient Positioning

The patient is placed supine on the operating table. Extended IV tubing and ventilator circuitry is employed so that the patient may be turned 180 degrees from the anesthesiologist. Hair is clipped around the surgical site so that plastic drapes may be applied to the patient's skin. Long-acting paralytic agents are avoided to allow intraoperative facial nerve monitoring. Facial nerve monitoring electrodes are placed in the orbicularis oris and orbicularis oculi to allow intraoperative nerve monitoring.

Incision

A large C-shaped incision is made within the hair-bearing skin from superior and lateral to the lateral orbital rim inferiorly into the neck overlying the sternocleido-

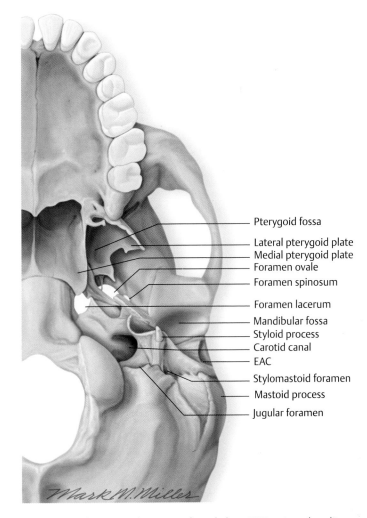

Fig. 11.4 Infratemporal anatomy from below. EAC, external auditory canal.

mastoid (SCM) muscle (**Fig. 11.8**). This incision extends to the level of the superficial layer of the deep temporal fascia. A horizontal incision is made down to bone at the level of the temporal line. A posterior periosteal incision is made from the temporal line to the mastoid tip. The plane of dissection extends to that of the level of the SCM. The anterior border of the SCM is identified and is the anterior limit of the dissection within the neck. The greater auricular nerve is identified and preserved (**Fig. 11.9**).

Blind Sac Closure of the Ear Canal

The periosteum of the mastoid cortex is stripped forward, exposing the external auditory canal (EAC). The EAC is transected at the level of the bony-cartilaginous junction. Further anterior dissection can be facilitated by dissecting the parotid fascia from the SCM to the preauricular area. The skin of the EAC is skeletonized and everted. The everted skin edges are then oversewn with interrupted 4-0 nylon sutures. An anteriorly based musculoperiosteal flap is then created from the soft tissue of the postauricular area to form a second layer of closure. This flap is secured to the parotid fascia with 3-0 Vicryl suture (**Fig. 11.10**).

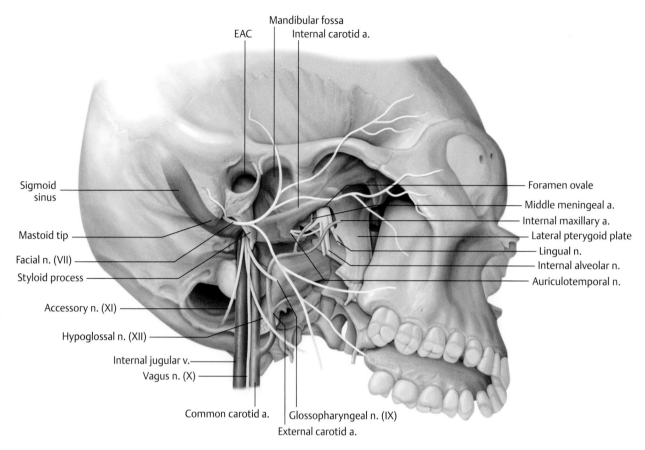

Fig. 11.5 Infratemporal neurovascular anatomy from a lateral view. EAC, external auditory canal.

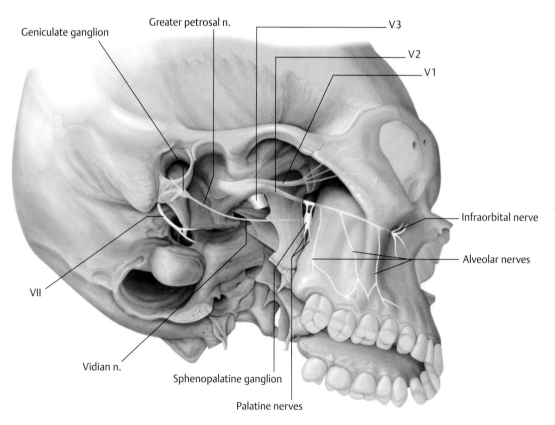

Fig. 11.6 Lateral infratemporal neuroanatomy deep to the pterygoid muscles.

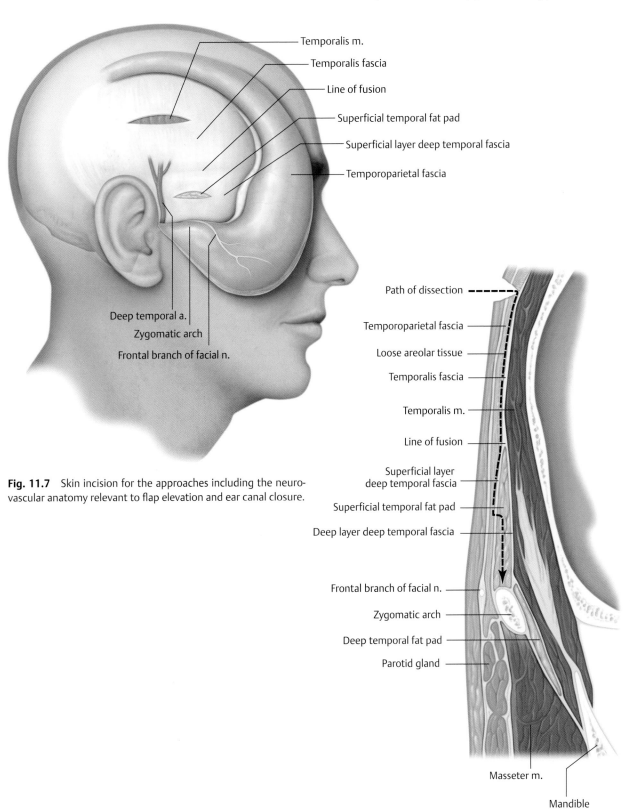

Fig. 11.7 Skin incision for the approaches including the neuro-vascular anatomy relevant to flap elevation and ear canal closure.

Fig. 11.8 Dissection plane for flap elevation, with attention to preservation of the frontal branch of the facial nerve. The nerve lies in the plane deep to the superficial temporal fascia and the superficial layer of the deep temporal fascia.

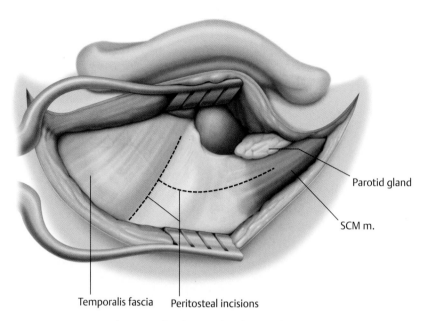

Fig. 11.9   Depiction of periosteal incisions. The incision along the linea temporalis extends to the zygomatic root. SCM, sternocleidomastoid.

Parotid Dissection

The anterior limit of the dissection is limited, in part, by the frontal branch of the facial nerve. To maximize exposure while preserving the frontal branch, it must be identified. This is most readily accomplished by identifying the frontal branch as it leaves the main trunk of the facial nerve. The main trunk of the facial nerve lie ap-

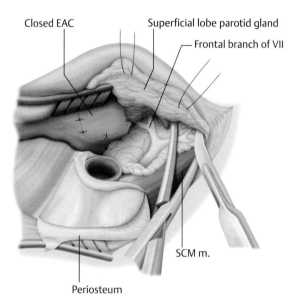

Fig. 11.10   Skin flap reflected forward, ear canal oversewn, and delineation of the intraparotid facial nerve. SCM, sternocleidomastoid.

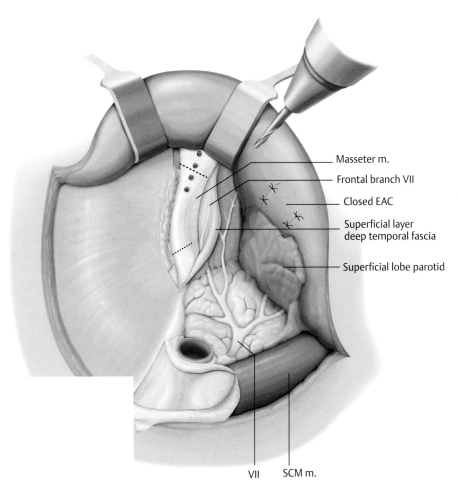

Masseter m.
Frontal branch VII
Closed EAC
Superficial layer
deep temporal fascia
Superficial lobe parotid

VII   SCM m.

Fig. 11.11 Completion of facial nerve exposure within the parotid, and preparation for zygomatic osteotomies. EAC, external auditory canal; SCM, sternocleidomastoid.

proximately 1 cm deep and 1 cm inferior to the tragal pointer in line with the tympanomastoid suture line. Once the main trunk has been identified, the frontal branch is traced to the periphery. The remaining branches of the facial nerve are not dissected (**Fig. 11.11**).

Temporalis Muscle and Zygomatic Arch Mobilization

To fully access the infratemporal fossa, the temporalis muscle must be completely mobilized. The zygomatic arch serves as the main barrier to the inferior mobilization of the temporalis muscle. The zygomatic arch therefore must be mobilized. The periosteum of the zygomatic arch is incised while retracting and protecting the frontal branch of the facial nerve. Titanium mini-plates are pre-plated to span the anterior and posterior osteotomies. The plates are then removed and the osteotomies are created. The zygomatic arch is left attached to the temporalis muscle. The entire temporalis muscle is dissected out of the temporal fossa, using an inferior to superior motion to transect the fibers sharply from their bony attachment. Great care is taken to preserve the blood supply and innervation of the muscle to prevent postoperative atrophy. The muscle is reflected inferiorly along with the zygomatic arch and left attached to the coronoid process (**Figs. 11.11 and 11.12**).

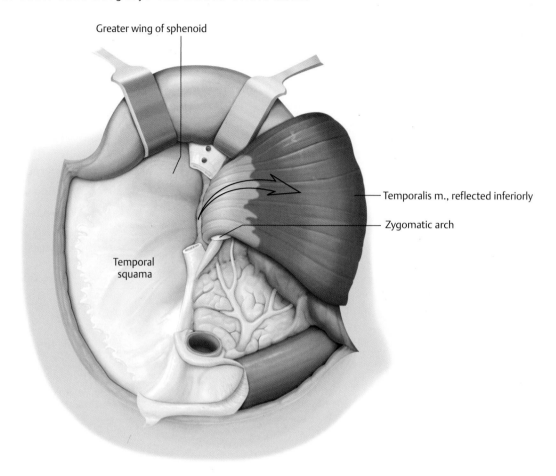

Greater wing of sphenoid

Temporalis m., reflected inferiorly

Zygomatic arch

Temporal squama

Fig. 11.12   Completion of zygomatic osteotomies and inferior reflection of the temporalis muscle, with exposure of the upper limit of the intratemporal fossa.

Subtotal Petrosectomy

A complete canal–wall–down mastoidectomy is performed, exenterating all air cell tracts (**Fig. 11.13**). Residual canal skin and the tympanic membrane are removed, along with the malleus and incus. The stapes is left undisturbed. The floor of the middle fossa is then decompressed. As the dissection is carried anteriorly, the glenoid fossa is removed. The eustachian tube is opened and the horizontal carotid artery is skeletonized. If indicated, the labyrinth and cochlea may be removed to improve exposure.

Intratemporal Fossa Exposure

The mandibular condyle is retracted inferiorly, along with the temporalis muscle and zygomatic arch (**Fig. 11.2**). Great care is taken to avoid stretching the frontal branch and main trunk of the facial nerve. The middle meningeal artery and mandibular branch of the trigeminal nerve (V3) may be divided to allow dissection into the infra-temporal fossa. The tensor tympani muscle is reflected out of its canal, and the bony eustachian tube is removed to its isthmus. Skeletonization and bony decompression of the middle fossa dura and carotid artery allow further exposure to the petrous apex and clivus (**Fig. 11.3**). If indicated, the carotid artery may be mobilized out of the carotid canal, providing free access to the petrous apex and clivus.

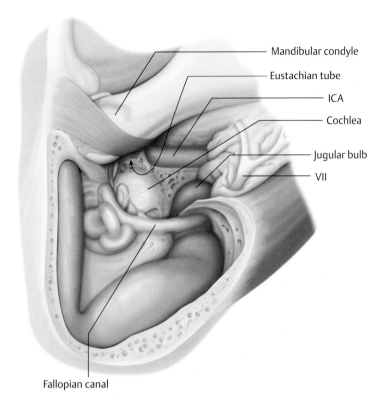

Mandibular condyle
Eustachian tube
ICA
Cochlea
Jugular bulb
VII

Fallopian canal

Fig. 11.13 Complete canal-wall–down exposure. The sigmoid sinus is skeletonized. The jugular bulb and vertical carotid artery are identified. Note the relationship of the internal carotid artery to the eustachian tube. ICA, internal carotid artery.

Extension into Nasopharynx or Cavernous Sinus (Type C Approach)

The lateral and medial pterygoid muscle are released from the attachments to the skull base and reflected inferiorly or removed. The mandibular and maxillary branches of the trigeminal nerve (V2 and V3) are transected. The pterygoid plates may then be resected. This allows further dissection of the membranous eustachian tube to the nasopharynx. The nasopharynx may then be fully exposed. The pterygoid plate and base of the greater wing of the sphenoid sinus may be removed to gain further exposure to the sphenoid sinus and cavernous sinus (**Fig. 11.3**).

Wound Closure

Type B

The defect left by the approach may be partially filled with a free abdominal fat graft. The vascularized temporalis muscle may then be rotated into the surgical defect for wound closure (**Fig. 11.14**). The skin is then closed in layers, a dependent drain is left in the wound, and a pressure dressing is applied.

Type C

The defect is closed much as in the type B approach. Careful attention is given to closure of the nasopharyngeal mucosa to prevent leakage of saliva into the wound. Because of this risk, the use of a free abdominal fat graft is discouraged (**Figs. 11.15 and 11.16**).

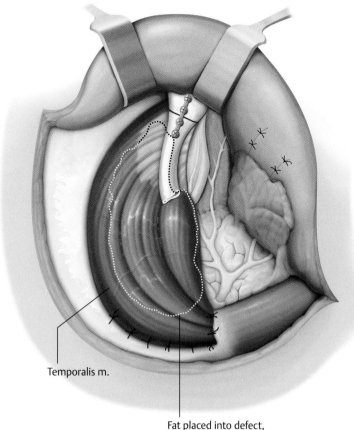

Temporalis m.

Fat placed into defect,
deep to temporalis m.

Fig. 11.14 Closure of the type B approach with anterior rotation of the temporalis muscle.

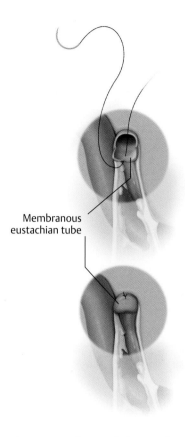

Membranous
eustachian tube

Fig. 11.15 Closure of the membranous eustachian tube to prevent cerebrospinal fluid (CSF) leak in the event of intradural dissection.

◆ Technical Pearls

- Type D modification: The Fisch D approach to the infratemporal fossa is a preauricular approach designed to approach lesions of the anterior infratemporal fossa, lateral orbital wall, and pterygopalatine fossa. Unlike in the Fisch B and C approaches, the middle ear and eustachian tube are not obliterated and conductive hearing is not sacrificed. Because the middle ear is spared, the petrous internal carotid artery is not fully exposed. The floor of the middle fossa may be drilled away in an extradural fashion to allow full access to the intratemporal fossa.
- Ear canal closure: Meticulous closure of the ear canal is necessary to prevent postoperative wound complications. This is particularly important if a cerebrospinal fluid leak is present.
- Free flaps: A microvascular free flap may be needed to close a large communication with the nasopharynx, particularly if there is a history of previous irradiation.
- Management of the stapes: In Fisch's description of these approaches, the stapes suprastructure was removed to prevent inadvertent injury to the stapes. We have found this manipulation of the stapes to be an unnecessary risk and have not had complications related to leaving the stapes intact.

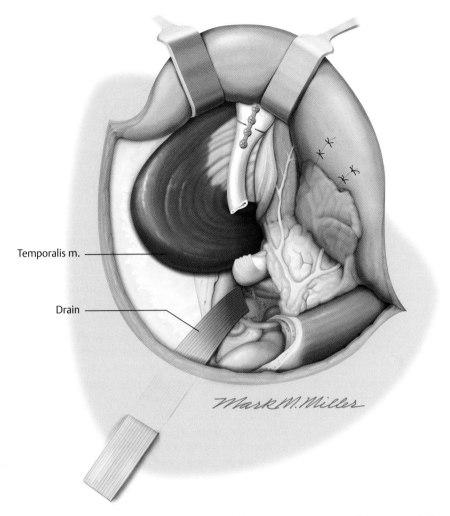

Fig. 11.16 Closure of the type C approach with deeper anterior rotation of the temporalis flap accompanied by closure of the nasopharyngeal mucosa.

◆ Conclusion

The Fisch infratemporal fossa approaches provide wide access to lesions of the jugular foramen, vertical and petrous carotid artery, the full extent of the infratemporal fossa, the pterygopalatine fossa, the clivus, the nasopharynx, and the cavernous sinus. This approach affords removal of large lesions affecting the lateral skull base and provides essential exposure to the neurovascular structures in this complex region.

Suggested Readings

Donald PJ. Infratemporal fossa: middle cranial fossa approach. In: Donald PJ, ed. Surgery of the Skull Base. Philadelphia: Lippincott-Raven, 1998:309–339

Fisch U, Mattox D. Microsurgery of the Skull Base. New York: Theime. 1988

House JW, Lin J, Friedman RA, Cullen RD. Translabyrinthine Approach Otologic Surgery, 3rd ed. Philadelphia: Saunders Elsevier, 2010: Chapter 46

12

The Preauricular Infratemporal Approach

Rick A. Friedman and James Lin

The preauricular infratemporal fossa (ITF) is not directly accessible owing to its lateral borders. In the last half-century surgeons have developed different surgical approaches to the IFTF with improved preservation of function and cosmesis. According to Conley's classification, lesions that occur in the IFTF may originate as a primary lesion in the IFTF or from any contiguous structures including the aerodigestive tract medially, the skull base and neural components superiorly, and the parotid gland laterally. Rarely, a malignancy from another site may metastasize to the IFTF. Because of the varying pathology that occurs in this region, the surgical approach is often tailored to the aggressiveness of the lesion, its extent, and the functional and cosmetic consequences. The preauricular IFTF approach is not suitable for lesions that involve the tympanic ring, jugular bulb, middle or inner ear, or lower cranial nerves.

For the purposes of this chapter, the preauricular IFTF is composed of the region inferior to the greater wing of the sphenoid and the temporal bone anterior to the tympanic ring (**Fig. 12.1**). This region includes the parapharyngeal space medially and the masticator space laterally; therefore, important contents of the preauricular IFTF include the carotid artery, cranial nerve V3, the internal maxillary artery, the eustachian tube, and the pterygoid venous plexus and muscles. The anterior border of the IFTF is the pterygoid muscles. The neurovascular foramina along the superior preauricular IFTF include the carotid canal, foramen ovale, foramen spinosum, and foramen lacerum. Its lateral borders include the parotid gland and facial nerve, the zygomatic arch, the mandible, and the temporalis and masseter muscles. Mobilizing the structures comprising the lateral border allows access to the preauricular infratemporal fossa.

◆ Preoperative Workup

The diagnosis of infratemporal fossa lesions is often delayed because they are rare and the region is poorly accessible for examination. Patients are more commonly referred from other physicians with radiologic studies in hand. Initially, a thorough history is taken and a physical examination is performed. Special attention is paid to the head and neck and the neurologic examination, especially of the cranial nerves. Varying degrees of facial hypesthesia may occur depending on the amount of trigeminal nerve involvement. Jaw deviation toward the affected side and temporalis wasting resulting from lateral pterygoid and temporalis muscle denervation may also be noted. Trismus secondary to irritation or fixation of masticatory muscles may also occur, which should prompt careful planning for securing the airway before surgery. Eustachian tube involvement may lead to serous otitis media and conductive hearing loss.

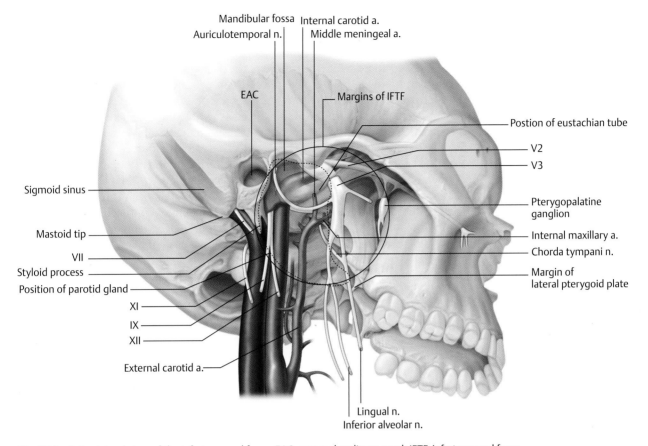

Mandibular fossa
Auriculotemperal n.
Internal carotid a.
Middle meningeal a.
EAC
Margins of IFTF
Postion of eustachian tube
V2
V3
Sigmoid sinus
Pterygopalatine ganglion
Mastoid tip
Internal maxillary a.
VII
Chorda tympani n.
Styloid process
Position of parotid gland
Margin of lateral pterygoid plate
XI
IX
XII
External carotid a.
Lingual n.
Inferior alveolar n.

Fig. 12.1   Inferolateral view of the infratemporal fossa. EAC, external auditory canal; IFTF, infratemporal fossa.

Radiographs provide a great deal of information regarding the nature and extent of the lesion. Both computed tomography (CT) and magnetic resonance imaging (MRI) are performed to evaluate the bony and soft tissue extent of the lesion in the IFTF in the axial and coronal planes. At least one of these imaging modalities should be contrasted. The radiologic characteristics of the tumor may be very suggestive of a pathologic diagnosis, but a tissue sample of the lesion may be necessary. Fine-needle aspiration under image guidance can yield cytologic specimen for diagnosis. Having a tissue diagnosis before the procedure allows the surgeon and patient to better understand the efficacy of surgical resection, the surgical margins required, and the overall prognosis. A pathologic diagnosis also guides the physician to seek adjuvant therapy and to perform a metastatic workup, if indicated.

If the tumor is highly vascular on imaging, then obtaining a biopsy of the lesion is ill-advised. Vasculature of the lesion can be studied with magnetic resonance angiography MRA and/or magnetic resonance venography (MRV) or conventional angiography. The benefit to performing true angiography is that it allows access for the interventional radiologist to embolize the tumor preoperatively, preferably within 48 to 72 hours of resection. If the lesion is amenable to resection and the carotid artery appears to be involved with tumor, then a temporary balloon occlusion (TBO) with xenon CT is performed to determine the risk of cerebral ischemia if the artery is occluded or partially resected. Once the nature and extent of the tumor are determined, a neurosurgeon and possibly a reconstructive surgeon are involved in the operative planning.

◆ Surgical Technique

The patient shampoos for 3 nights preoperatively with PHisoHex shampoo. On the day of the operation, a generous shave of the ipsilateral hemicranium is traditionally performed; however, for the sake of cosmesis, a 1-cm strip of hair may instead be removed over the planned incision site. After anesthesia is induced, the neurosurgeon may place a lumbar drain if dural involvement with tumor is noted. The patient is then positioned supine on the operating table with the head placed in pins or a Mayfield head rest, angled 45 degrees away. Electrodes for monitoring of the facial nerve are placed into the orbicularis muscles. If the internal carotid artery is to be mobilized or resected, somatosensory evoked potentials are monitored. The patient undergoes placement of sequential compression devices, a Foley catheter, and an orogastric tube. The anesthesiologist may administer Decadron, mannitol, and/or furosemide if extensive temporal lobe retraction is anticipated. If prolonged temporal lobe retraction or brain parenchyma is expected to be dissected, a dose of phenytoin is given. The patient also receives a dose of IV antibiotics with good cerebrospinal fluid (CSF) penetration such as cefuroxime prior to incision. In patients with cephalosporin or penicillin allergies, vancomycin is the preferred alternative. One percent lidocaine with epinephrine (1:100,000) is injected into the planned incision, and the patient's ipsilateral hemicranium, neck, and potential donor sites for reconstruction (e.g., abdomen) are prepped and draped. All prepped areas are subsequently covered with Ioban.

The minimum incision planned is a hemicoronal incision with the inferior border extending just anterior to the tragus. If a neck dissection or exploration is planned, the inferior limb of the incision is designed as a Blair-type incision with extension

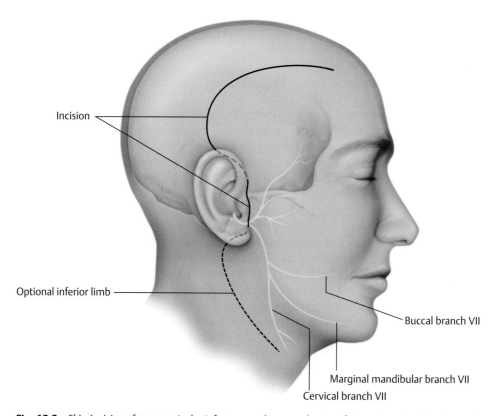

Fig. 12.2 Skin incisions for preauricular infratemporal approach. An inferior extension into the neck provides control of the great vessels when necessary.

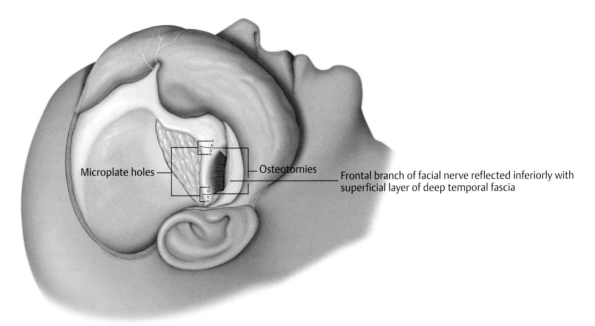

Microplate holes —   — Osteotomies   — Frontal branch of facial nerve reflected inferiorly with
superficial layer of deep temporal fascia

Fig. 12.3 The cutaneous flap is elevated to the orbital rim and malar eminence. The plane of dissection shifts at the upper lateral orbital rim from deep to the superficial temporal fascia to deep to the superficial layer of the deep temporal fascia. This affords protection of the frontal branch of the facial nerve. Microplate holes are drilled prior to zygomatic osteotomies.

into a cervical crease (**Fig. 12.2**). The deepest portion of the incision is made superiorly above the temporalis muscles down to bone. The flap is subsequently raised in a subpericranial plane and brought over the temporalis fascia. At the area of the temporal fat pad, the fascia of the muscle splits into a superficial and deep layer, around the fat pad, attaching to the lateral and medial aspects of the zygomatic arch, respectively. The frontal branch of the facial nerve travels within or just deep to the temporoparietal fascia at the level of the superior orbital rim. To protect this nerve branch, the plane of dissection should be transitioned just deep to the superficial layer of the deep temporalis fascia (**Fig. 12.3**) at the level of the temporal fat pad. Following this plane brings the surgeon to the zygomatic arch, which is freed of its periosteum on its medial and lateral borders with an elevator. Anteriorly, the dissection plane is continued to expose the superior orbital rim and its transition to the anterior attachment of the zygomatic arch. The frontal and trochlear branches exiting their foramina superior to the orbit are identified.

If a full incision involving the neck is involved, the flap on the face and neck are raised just superficial to the parotid-masseteric fascial and subplatysmal planes, respectively. At this point, a neck exploration can be performed, and the external and internal carotid artery, internal jugular vein, and cranial nerves X to XII are identified and tagged.

Once the skin and facial flap is raised, the parotid gland is freed from the masseter muscle bluntly. In preparation for transposition of the zygomatic arch, the masseter and temporalis attachments to the arch are freed anteriorly with electrocautery. Titanium microplates are fixed across osteotomy sites with screws and then removed. The osteotomies are subsequently made and the arch swung inferiorly pedicled on the masseter muscle. The temporalis muscle is detached from its superior attachments, leaving a cuff of fascia superiorly for reattachment after the procedure. The muscle is dissected free from the temporal fossa and also swung inferiorly, attached to its blood supply and the coronoid process. As the temporalis muscle is freed from its bony fossa, the infratemporal crest should be visualized (**Fig. 12.4**).

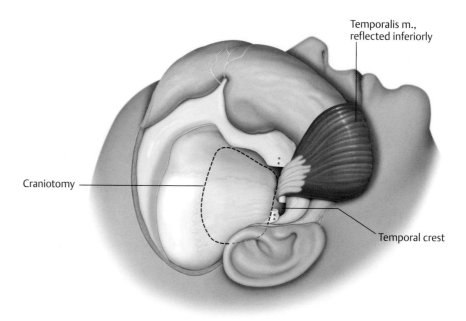

Fig. 12.4 Temporalis muscle is elevated from the temporal fossa. Zygomatic osteotomies allow greater inferior reflection of the muscle, providing an enhanced view of the infratemporal fossa.

At this point, the surgeon may improve exposure prior to the craniotomy with an armamentarium of maneuvers. To allow greater soft tissue displacement, a Blair-type extension is made, and the main trunk of the facial nerve is identified exiting the stylomastoid foramen. If the soft tissue attachments along the posterior edge of the parotid gland and around the facial nerve are transected, leaving a cuff of tissue around the facial nerve, the parotid gland can be further mobilized from its underlying attachments and the mandible can be inferiorly displaced. Mobilizing the mandible requires comprehensive electrocautery dissection of the masseter from its origin, division of the stylomandibular and sphenomandibular ligaments, and dislocating the glenoid fossa inferiorly. Further exposure may be achieved by resecting the mandibular condyle or fracturing the coronoid process to allow a greater range of motion for the pedicled temporalis muscle. In performing any of these maneuvers, care must be taken to preserve the blood supply of the muscle originating from the internal maxillary artery, just medial to the mandibular condyle and coronoid process.

With the temporal crest in view, the inferior skull base may be exposed medially in a subperiosteal plane to expose the lateral pterygoid plate anteriorly, V3, and the foramen spinosum posteriorly. A frontotemporal craniotomy is then performed from the pterion anteriorly to a region just superior to the glenoid fossa posteriorly using high-speed burs to outline the bone flap. If the temporal bone is extensively pneumatized, air cell tracts may be encountered posteroinferiorly that require bone wax occlusion. Once the bone flap is freed from its lateral attachments, it is freed from its underlying dura with an Adson periosteal elevator, or "joker" (**Fig. 12.5**).

Under a microscope, the dura of the temporal lobe is elevated from the middle cranial fossa floor with an elevator. A lumbar drain may be opened or the aforementioned medications may be administered to relax the brain at this time. We prefer to begin the elevation posteriorly to identify the petrous ridge and arcuate eminence. The middle meningeal artery and V3 are encountered initially anteriorly and laterally. The greater superficial petrosal nerve is then encountered more medially and posteriorly. A few more maneuvers can be performed to improve exposure of the

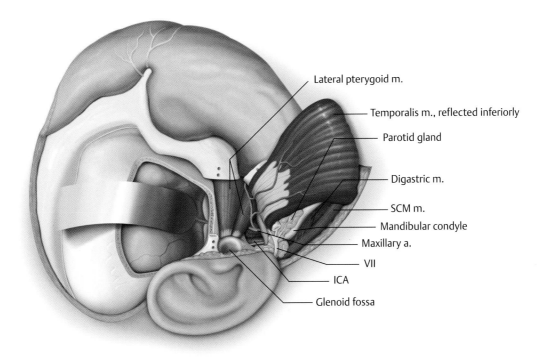

Fig. 12.5 Craniotomy completed, temporal lobe extradural retractor in place. The floor of the middle fossa is still intact. ICA, internal carotid artery; SCM, sternocleidomastoid.

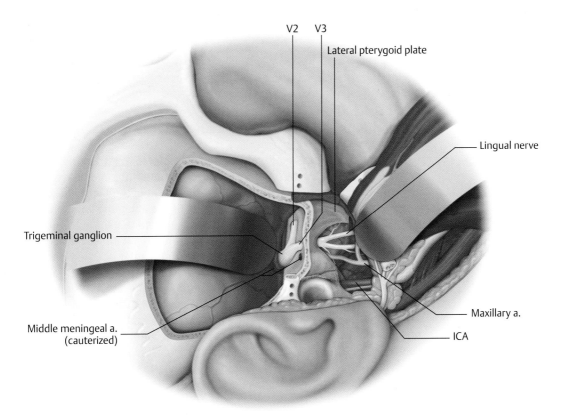

Fig. 12.6 Dissection of the pterygoid muscles providing a view of the deep neurovascular structures. ICA, internal carotid artery.

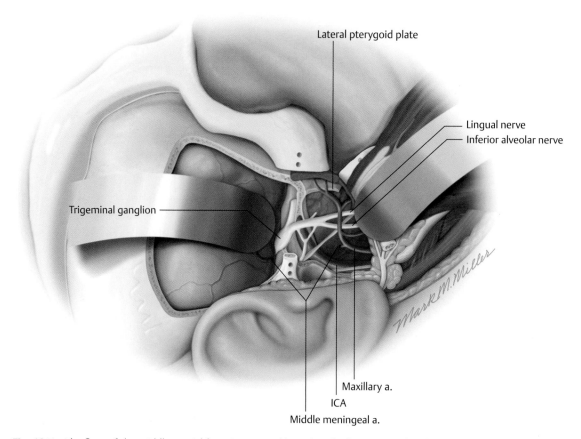

Fig. 12.7   The floor of the middle cranial fossa is removed lateral to the foramen ovale. The middle meningeal artery is sectioned at the foramen spinosum. Dissection can extend anteromedial to the cochlea for exposure of the eustachian tube and ultimately the horizontal segment of the petrous carotid artery. ICA, internal carotid artery.

skull base: the middle meningeal artery is coagulated and ligated, and the dural envelopment around V3 may be sharply dissected away from the nerve using a beaver blade (**Fig. 12.6**).

At this point, the self-retaining retractors are placed to retract the temporal lobe. A high-speed drill is used to perform a craniectomy of the middle cranial fossa floor. The extent of bony removal is dictated by the extent of tumor. In general, the craniectomy can be brought to the level of V3 medially, opening the foramen ovale laterally (**Fig. 12.6**). This nerve branch can be worked around to expose the eustachian tube and internal carotid artery (ICA) periosteum. Once the ICA is identified in its petrous route, it is carefully followed using diamond burs anteriorly and posteriorly. At its genu, it is traced inferiorly to its vertical segment in the infratemporal fossa (**Fig. 12.7**). In selected cases, V3 may be cut to improve exposure. Anteriorly, bony removal can be extended to the foramen rotundum, superior orbital fissure, and optic canal. Throughout the dissection, bleeding may occur inferiorly from the pterygoid plexus of veins and from the communicating vessels around V3. This bleeding is typically controlled with bipolar cautery and/or gently packing with Surgicel. Care must be taken to prevent disruption of the temporalis muscle's blood supply, as it often serves as the reconstructive flap at the end of the procedure.

Once the tumor is adequately exposed, tumor removal proceeds. A partial mandibulectomy may be necessary, the parotid gland may be removed in its entirety, and portions of the pterygoid musculature and trigeminal nerve resected. Dura and involved brain parenchyma may also be included in the resection if it is felt by the surgeon to be indicated. Tumor around the ICA may be carefully dissected away. In some cases, an involved portion of the ICA may be resected if acceptable risk is noted on preoperative balloon occlusion studies.

With the tumor removed, reconstruction can begin. If dura has been opened, it can be closed with the aid of temporalis fascia, acellular dermis, or synthetic dural replacement such as Duragen. The distal eustachian tube is packed and oversewn. The bone flap from the middle cranial fossa craniotomy is replaced and fixed with miniplates. A significant amount of dead space results along the inferior craniectomy and within the infratemporal fossa. This space should be obliterated with vascularized tissue, especially if there is communication with the aerodigestive tract. If the temporalis muscle is viable, the muscle may be divided vertically into two pedicles. The anterior portion may be placed into the inferior wound defect while the posterior portion is swung into the anterior temporal fossa and sewn to its remaining fascial cuff. If the defect is too large for the available temporalis muscle or the temporalis muscle is not viable, a microvascular free flap such as a rectus abdominis flap is the preferred method of reconstruction. If the dead space obliteration allows, the zygomatic arch can be replaced and fixed with its pre-fitted miniplates. A Penrose drain may be placed deep into the wound, and closure is performed in layers using inverted, interrupted 3–0 Vicryl sutures followed by a running, locked skin closure with 3–0 Prolene or nylon suture. A pressure dressing may be placed, but only if there is little risk of vascular compromise of the reconstruction.

◆ Postoperative Care

The patient is transferred from the operating room to the intensive care unit for close neurologic observation and is allowed to awaken from anesthesia. Intravenous antibiotics are continued for a total of 24 hours perioperatively. The patient may be allowed ice chips on postoperative day 1 with the diet increased afterward as tolerated. Isotonic IV fluids are administered until oral intake is adequate. Provided there are no complications, the arterial line and urinary catheter are removed on postoperative day 1 and the patient is transferred to the floor. A dressing, if placed, is kept until postoperative day 3. A lumbar drain may be continued postoperatively, if there has been significant dural resection, at a rate tolerable by the patient for 3 to 5 days. After this time period, the drain is clamped for 24 hours and removed if no CSF leak occurs. At 2 weeks, the patient is initiated on jaw exercises to prevent trismus.

◆ Complications and Adverse Outcomes

Perhaps the most feared intraoperative event is damage to the internal carotid artery. As discussed above, the probability of ICA manipulation should be determined by preoperative imaging, and the likelihood of cerebral ischemia resulting from loss of the ipsilateral carotid determined by temporary balloon occlusion with xenon CT. Resection or inadvertent damage to the ICA requires the aid of a neurosurgeon for management. The carotid may be repaired, grafted, or bypassed if preoperative studies determine that the probability of cerebral ischemia is high. Postoperatively, the patient requires close neurologic observation and management of blood pressure, preferably by an intensivist accustomed to dealing with neurosurgical patients. Other intraoperative bleeding is more readily controlled with bipolar cautery or packing with Surgicel or Gelfoam.

In the immediate postoperative period, postoperative intracranial hemorrhage may occur, leading to altered sensorium, blood pressure fluctuations, or acute anisocoria. If these symptoms progress rapidly in the immediate postoperative period, the patient may be rushed to the operating room for wound exploration, evacuation of blood clot, and control of bleeding vessels. If the symptomatology is less clear, the patient may undergo emergency noncontrasted head CT to search for intracranial hemorrhage, followed by possible operative evacuation of a hematoma.

While raising the scalp flap, transection or traction injury to several nerves may occur. The frontal branch of the facial nerve may be damaged, resulting in a weak forehead if the scalp flap is raised too superficially; this is avoided with the measures described above. The main trunk of the facial nerve may be damaged with traction in an attempt to mobilize the parotid gland; this may be avoided by leaving a cuff of tissue around the nerve between the stylomastoid foramen and the parotid gland and decreasing the tension placed on the nerve by retractors. Anesthesia of the forehead and scalp are likely to occur from the incision or traction on the supratrochlear and supraorbital nerves.

A cosmetic deformity may result from atrophy or loss of the temporalis muscle attached to the anterior temporal fossa. Temporomandibular joint dysfunction resulting from inferior displacement of the mandible may occur, and some authorities advocate consistent condylar resection as a less morbid alternative. Physical therapy and jaw exercises may help decrease the functional deficits. Prolonged traction on the temporal lobe may lead to edema with resultant speech deficit and/or seizures. These problems are treated with steroids and an anticonvulsant such as phenytoin. Dissection along or sacrifice of V2 and V3 may lead to anesthesia or neuropathic pain of the face and tongue and weakness of the ipsilateral masticatory muscles.

A postoperative CSF wound leak or CSF rhinorrhea may occur if there is dural resection. Prevention is the best strategy in managing this problem with watertight dural closure, ample eustachian tube packing and closure, and layered watertight wound closure. If the dural resection is significant, maintaining the lumbar drain postoperatively helps decrease CSF pressure while allowing the dura and wound to partially heal closed. Wound leaks that occur postoperatively are initially managed with bed rest, a pressure dressing, and wound overclosure with 0-silk or 0-nylon sutures. A lumbar drain may be inserted in the postoperative period to divert CSF away from the leak site. CSF rhinorrhea is initially managed by lumbar drainage for 3 days and bed rest. These conservative measures control the majority of CSF leaks, but if they fail, the wound may require reexploration and additional closure of the eustachian tube, dura, and/or wound.

Wound infection is a rare complication in these cases and is usually prevented with careful preoperative preparation of the operative site and perioperative antibiotics. In the rare case that an infection does occur, it is treated aggressively with IV antibiotics, as an infection potentially may lead to wound breakdown and spread of infection intracranially. Intracranial infections unrelated to wound infection may also occur in the postoperative setting. Those patients who note worsening of headache, fever, chills, altered sensorium, or stiff neck receive IV antibiotics without hesitation. A head CT scan is then performed prior to examination of CSF for evidence of meningitis. If a localized intracranial infection is still suspected, a contrasted MRI is obtained to identify epidural, subdural, or parenchymal abscess. The treatment of meningitis is intravenous antibiotics and possibly steroids, with the duration dependent on the patient's symptoms and findings at repeat CSF examination. The treatment of intracranial abscess includes surgical drainage and intravenous antibiotics for several weeks.

◆ Conclusion

The preauricular infratemporal approach provides excellent access to the contents of the infratemporal fossa from above. The addition of the craniectomy of the floor of the middle fossa allows dissection of tumors that dumbbell through the foramen ovale, such as trigeminal neuromas. The advantage of the approach from above is minimal risk of morbidity to the facial nerve and no postoperative hearing loss.

Suggested Readings

Leonetti JP, Anderson DE, Marzo SJ, Origitano TC, Schuman R. The preauricular subtemporal approach for transcranial petrous apex tumors. Otol Neurotol 2008;29:380–383

Mansour OI, Carrau RL, Snyderman CH, Kassam AB. Preauricular infratemporal fossa surgical approach: modifications of the technique and surgical indications. Skull Base 2004;14:143–151, discussion 151

13

Temporal Bone Resection

Antonio De la Cruz and James Lin

Temporal bone malignancies arise from different areas: primary from the external ear canal, primary from the middle ear space or mastoid, and secondary from adjacent structures such as the pinna or parotid gland. Primary malignancy of the temporal bone is uncommon, with squamous cell carcinoma being the most common type. As a result of its rarity and lack of uniformity in staging and treatment, an evidence-based multidisciplinary protocol for management of the disease remains elusive. Surgery is the mainstay for cure.

The surgical treatment of temporal bone malignancy has evolved over the past several decades. Earlier attempts to control disease involved mastoidectomy with planned postoperative radiotherapy. Later attempts to achieve better disease control involved en-bloc resection of the temporal bone. There remains controversy among authors regarding the extent of resection necessary to improve 5-year survival while being mindful of quality of life, but there is a common theme of at least en-bloc resection of the lateral temporal bone with added removal of grossly involved medial regions. The surgical goal is negative margins upon completion of the procedure.

◆ Preoperative Workup

Initial evaluation begins with a thorough history and physical examination. Otorrhea, ear pain, and bleeding are the classic triad of symptoms of temporal bone squamous cell carcinoma. These symptoms and a suspicious lesion on examination warrant a biopsy to confirm the diagnosis of malignancy. An audiogram is performed. Radiographic evaluation is used to determine the extent of disease with high-resolution computed tomography (CT) scanning complemented by magnetic resonance imaging (MRI). CT provides excellent bony detail of erosion, whereas MRI provides more soft tissue detail. At least one of these modalities should include a contrasted examination of the neck to identify regional nodal metastases. An otolaryngologist is central to the treatment of temporal bone malignancy, whereas a head and neck surgeon and a neurosurgeon may be consulted for extratemporal and intracranial extension of tumor, respectively. A chest radiograph and liver function testing are performed to rule out distant metastases. From the physical exam and radiographs, the stage of the tumor may be determined; the authors prefer the system described by Arriaga et al and later modified by Moody et al (**Table 13.1**).

One controversy is whether to resect the internal carotid artery (ICA) to obtain adequate cancer margins. If any manipulation of the ICA is expected, the patient undergoes temporary balloon occlusion with a complementary xenon CT scan to attempt to determine the risk of neurologic deficit with carotid resection. Cerebrovascular studies should demonstrate the patency of the circle of Willis with residual pressure and should also include the venous drainage of the brain, especially in the case where the ipsilateral venous sinuses appear to be involved with tumor and require resection. Patients with poor contralateral drainage may be at risk of venous infarction. Resection of involved dura and brain parenchyma, albeit controversial, may be performed.

Table 13.1 Pittsburgh Staging System for Temporal Bone Carcinoma

Status	Description
T1	Tumor limited to external auditory canal (EAC) without bony erosion or soft tissue extension
T2	Tumor with limited EAC bony erosion (not full thickness [FT]) or limited (<0.5 cm) soft tissue involvement
T3	Full-thickness erosion of EAC with limited (<0.5 cm) soft tissue involvement, or mastoid/ME involvement
T4	Involvement of cochlea, petrous apex, medial wall of the middle ear (ME), carotid canal, jugular foramen or dura, or >0.5 cm soft tissue involvement; facial paralysis

Source: From Moody SA, Hirsch BE, Myers EN. Squamous cell carcinoma of the external auditory canal: an evaluation of a staging system. Am J Otol. 2000;21(4):582–588. Reprinted by permission.

Finally, involvement of the jugular foramen and lower cranial nerves should prompt the treating physician to counsel the patient regarding swallowing deficits and potential rehabilitative measures.

Once a resection plan has been formed, a reconstructive surgeon familiar with skull base and cranial defects is involved in planning the wound closure. It is important not to compromise oncologic principles of tumor removal in an attempt to improve reconstructive outcomes. It is, however, reasonable to modify the handling of uninvolved soft tissues, blood vessels, and nerves in a manner that does not "burn any bridges" for the reconstructing surgeon.

◆ Surgical Technique

Skin Incision

A generous shave is performed of the hemicranium and neck. A spinal drain may be placed to decrease the risk of cerebrospinal fluid (CSF) wound leak if dural involvement is expected. An antibiotic with good CSF penetration is administered and maintained for 24 hours. If brain retraction is expected, mannitol, Decadron, and furosemide may be given at the beginning of surgery. Brain parenchyma dissection requires intravenous administration of an anticonvulsant such as phenytoin. The patient is placed supine on the operating room table with the head turned away. If a neck dissection is to be performed, a shoulder role may be placed for slight neck extension. Electrodes are placed in the orbicularis muscles for facial nerve monitoring. If surgical exploration of the jugular foramen is foreseen, neurophysiologic monitoring of the lower cranial nerves can also be performed. The operative site, including the neck, face, and ipsilateral hemicranium, is prepped and draped. Other sites of the body may be prepped and draped for reconstructive purposes.

A C-shaped incision is made 3 to 4 cm behind the postauricular crease, curving to the mastoid tip inferiorly and superiorly, anterior to the tragus. Further extensions of the incision may be necessary anteriorly or inferiorly if infratemporal fossa or neck dissection is planned, respectively. The lateral external auditory canal (EAC) must be separated from the skin flap, requiring a separate incision encompassing the lateral EAC. If the tumor is confined medially, a separate circumferential incision outlining a portion of the conchal bowl and tragus may be made (**Fig. 13.1**). If a wider, more lateral tumor margin is required, this circumferential incision may be connected to the

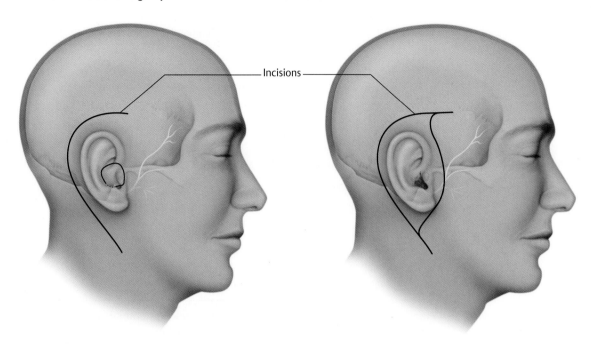

Incisions

Fig. 13.1　Standard incision for temporal bone resection.

Fig. 13.2　Standard incision for temporal bone resection requiring a pinna removal.

postauricular incision to encompass the entire pinna within the resection (**Fig. 13.2**). The inferior limb of the incision may be extended into the neck a variable amount depending on whether control of the great vessels and lower cranial nerves is desired or a neck dissection is to be performed.

Initially, the postauricular flap is raised anteriorly at a level superficial to the temporalis fascia and periosteum. Great care is taken to maintain negative margins while raising this flap. In order for flap elevation to continue anteriorly, the attachment of the skin flap to the ear canal must be crossed. This is accomplished by deepening the circumferential EAC incision until it is continuous with the plane of flap elevation. Frozen sections from the lateral margins on the scalp and facial flap, not from the tumor specimen, are sent to the pathology laboratory. The lateral EAC is oversewn. The flap is carried further anteriorly superficial to the parotid gland, to the anterior edge of the gland. The point at which the temporalis muscle and periosteum are incised to the bone depends on the lateral extent of the tumor and the margin desired. An attempt to stagger this deep incision from the skin incision should be made to facilitate a multilayer closure at the end of the procedure to decrease the risk of CSF fistula. The sternocleidomastoid muscle is detached from the mastoid tip anteriorly and reflected posteriorly to allow access to the posterior digastric and stylomastoid foramen.

Lateral Temporal Bone Resection: Indications

A lateral temporal bone resection is used for tumors lateral to the tympanic membrane without involvement of the mastoid. The completed resection has the medial border (from posterior to anterior) of thin bone overlying the sigmoid sinus and posterior fossa dura, the bony labyrinth and facial nerve, the medial wall of the middle ear with promontory and stapes suprastructure intact, and the deep lobe of the parotid gland with overlying facial nerve branches if superficial parotidectomy is performed. The superior border is the mastoid and middle ear tegmen; the inferior border is composed of the infratemporal fossa. The anterior border is variable and ranges from the temporomandibular joint (TMJ) periosteum to the infratemporal fossa, depending on tumor extension.

Lateral Temporal Bone Resection: Procedure

A wide cortical mastoidectomy is performed with high-speed drills. The mastoid tegmen, posterior fossa dura, and sigmoid sinus are skeletonized. The vertical facial nerve is identified by visualization of its epineural vessels through thinned bone. The facial nerve is followed down to the stylomastoid foramen at which a fibrous sheath around the nerve is encountered. It is best not to dissect the nerve out of this sheath, as attempts to do so will likely compromise its blood supply and result in facial paresis. The lateral and posterior semicircular canals are carefully skeletonized. The infralabyrinthine, retrofacial air cell tract is drilled medially. The bony external auditory canal is thinned, avoiding violation of the tumor. An extended facial recess is opened using a 1.5-mm diamond bur and extended inferiorly between the tympanic annulus and the facial nerve. The chorda tympani is sharply sectioned with this inferior extension (**Fig. 13.3**).

The facial recess is extended anteroinferiorly, following the tympanic annulus; care must be taken to identify a high or lateral jugular bulb. This dissection is brought forward to the anterior wall of the mastoid tip, to the mandibular periosteum. Superiorly, the middle fossa floor is followed anteriorly into the zygomatic root, "hugging" the bony external auditory canal (**Fig. 13.4**). The limit of this dissection is the TMJ periosteum (**Fig. 13.5**). Through the facial recess, the incudostapedial joint is then separated with a small hook or joint knife and the tendon of the tensor tympani is

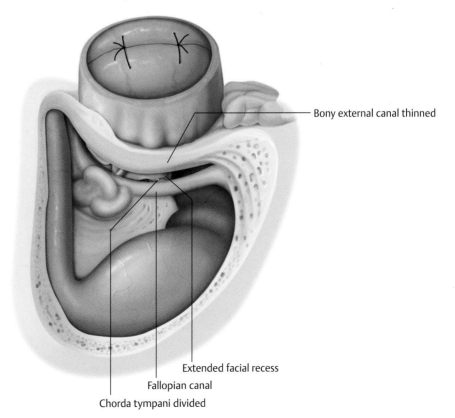

Bony external canal thinned

Extended facial recess

Fallopian canal

Chorda tympani divided

Fig. 13.3 The bony ear canal is closed, a mastoidectomy has been performed, and the facial recess has been extended.

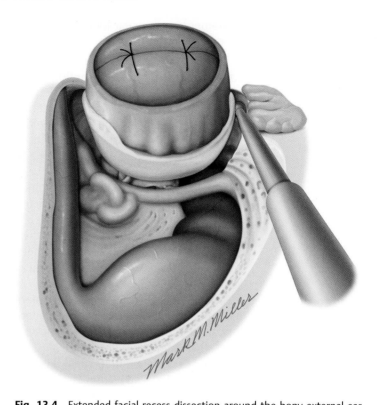

Fig. 13.4   Extended facial recess dissection around the bony external ear canal.

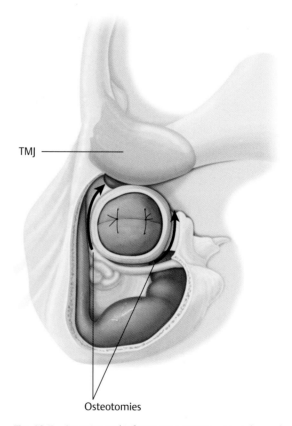

Fig. 13.5   Superior and inferior osteotomies are performed into the temporomandibular joint (TMJ).

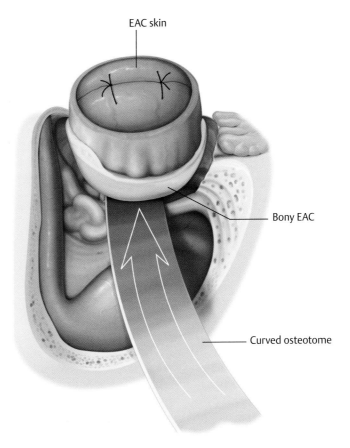

EAC skin

Bony EAC

Curved osteotome

Fig. 13.6 Osteotomy medial to tympanic membrane and lateral to carotid artery. EAC, external auditory canal.

cut. The EAC remains attached to the anteromedial middle ear cavity by the bone just lateral to the eustachian tube. A curved osteotome passed through the facial recess facilitates the detachment of the bony EAC. Care must be exercised with this maneuver as the carotid artery and facial nerve lie just medial to the osteotome (**Fig. 13.6**).

At the stylomastoid foramen, the main trunk of the facial nerve has been previously identified and a superficial parotidectomy may be performed. If the parotid is removed, it is left attached to the anterior EAC and removed en bloc.

When the tumor involves the anterior EAC, the dissection may include a portion of the mandibular condyle, which is removed using a reciprocating saw. Care is taken not to traumatize the internal maxillary artery, which lies deep to the mandible (**Fig. 13.7**).

Lateral Temporal Bone Resection: Reconstruction

The reconstruction of the lateral temporal bone resection defect depends on the extent of the tumor and if the area has been or will be radiated. A tumor confined to the EAC (T1) carries an excellent prognosis with primary surgical resection alone; radiation therapy is of little added benefit. In this case, a radical mastoidectomy cavity with a large meatoplasty can be created by lining the defect with a skin graft. The patient may benefit from a type III tympanoplasty with this simple reconstruction. If the patient continues to have a significant conductive hearing loss in the future, a formal ossicular reconstruction with cartilage blocks may be performed 1 year later.

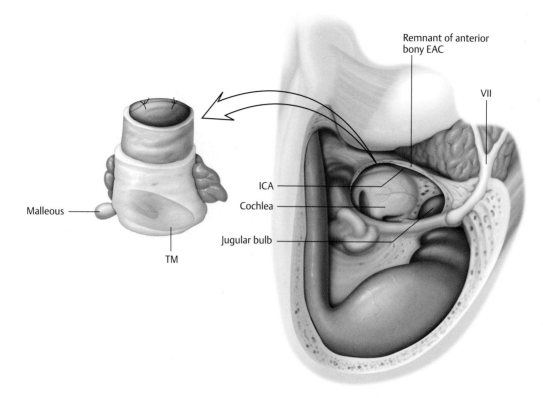

Fig. 13.7   Tumor specimen removed with the resultant cavity. EAC, external auditory canal; ICA, internal carotid artery; TM, tympanic membrane.

If the patient's tumor has received or will receive radiation therapy to the operative site, covering the operative site with vascularized tissue is indicated. A local temporalis muscle flap can be placed into the defect with a skin graft to completely line the site of the EAC (**Fig. 13.8**).

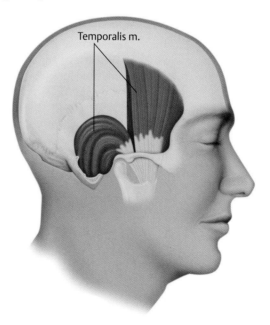

Fig. 13.8   A localized muscle flap is used to line the mastoid defect.

Subtotal Temporal Bone Resection: Indications

Subtotal temporal bone resection is the surgical therapy of choice for tumors medial to the tympanic membrane, into the mastoid, or involving the facial nerve. There is a core resection in this procedure with further extensions that are performed depending on the tumor's extent. The subtotal temporal bone resection deficit includes a medial border of (from posterior to anterior) sigmoid sinus and posterior fossa dura, internal auditory canal dura, the anterior petrous apex, and the vertical segment of the ICA. The anterior border is the TMJ periosteum. The inferior border is the jugular bulb, skull base periosteum, and a drilled-down vaginal process between the jugular bulb and ICA. The superior border is the middle fossa dura.

Subtotal Temporal Bone Resection: Procedure

A lateral temporal bone resection is performed. Bone overlying the sigmoid sinus and the middle and posterior fossa dura is removed using large diamond burs. Similar to performing a translabyrinthine craniotomy for acoustic neuroma, it is useful to extend the dural decompression a few centimeters posterior to the sigmoid sinus to facilitate access to more medial structures. Bone flakes along the dura may be sent to the pathology laboratory as a medial margin of the specimen. A labyrinthectomy is performed using a medium-sized bur (3 or 4 mm). The bony removal must be extended to decompress the most medial portions of the middle and posterior fossa dura down to the porus acusticus. Continuing dissection of the posterior semicircular canal inferiorly leads to the jugular bulb, which is skeletonized. The dura of the internal auditory canal is skeletonized (**Fig. 13.9**).

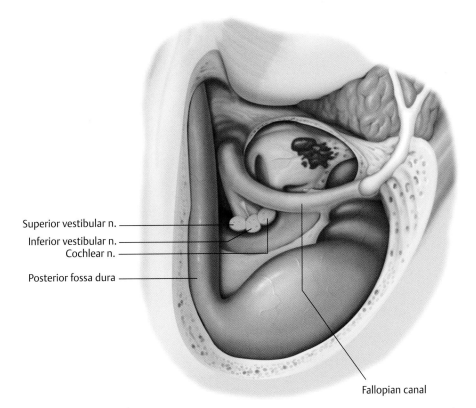

Superior vestibular n.
Inferior vestibular n.
Cochlear n.
Posterior fossa dura
Fallopian canal

Fig. 13.9 The internal auditory canal is skeletonized, with section of the cochlear and vestibular nerves.

Facial Nerve

The surgeon may choose to remove a portion of the facial nerve, especially if a preoperative or intraoperative examination indicates its involvement by tumor. The internal auditory canal (IAC) dura may be opened and the facial nerve resected along with the vestibular and cochlear nerve until negative margins are reached. The distal end of the nerve may be tagged and cut at the main trunk proximal to the pes anserinus if the tumor is primarily intratemporal. Alternatively, the individual branches may be identified, tagged, and cut more distally if the tumor involves the parotid gland. In either case, frozen sections from the distal nerve end(s) are sent to the pathology laboratory. The nerve may be cable grafted if margins are free of tumor (see below). When dealing with the facial nerve, the surgeon should consider the patient's quality of life with a facial nerve paralysis in light of the realistic chance for cure.

If the facial nerve is grossly uninvolved, it may be mobilized from the fallopian canal to access more medial structures. The nerve is skeletonized using small to medium-sized diamond burs applied parallel to the nerve through the labyrinthine, geniculate, horizontal, and vertical segments to the fibrous cuff at the stylomastoid foramen. The greater superficial petrosal nerve is also exposed anteromedial to the geniculate ganglion and sharply divided. The dura of the IAC is opened and the nerve freed proximally toward the cerebellopontine angle (CPA). The thin remnant of fallopian canal bone overlying the nerve is removed with a fine dissecting instrument, and the nerve is subsequently rerouted posteriorly (**Fig. 13.10**). Mobilization of the nerve may result in temporary facial paresis (House-Brackmann grade 3 or 4).

With the facial nerve displaced from the fallopian canal, the remaining inferior tympanic ring and bone lateral to the jugular bulb is removed, and the periosteum overlying the carotid artery is identified carefully with a diamond bur and followed anterosuperiorly. All bone of the skull base inferior and lateral to the vaginal process separating the jugular bulb and proximal carotid artery is drilled to skull base perios-

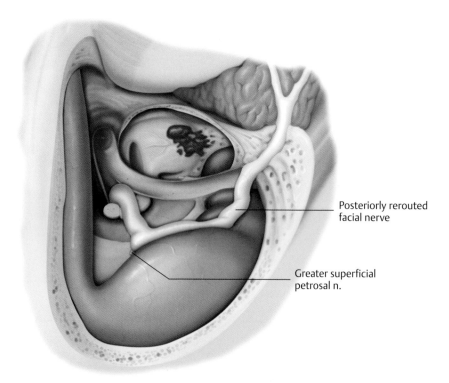

Posteriorly rerouted facial nerve

Greater superficial petrosal n.

Fig. 13.10   Mobilization of the facial nerve posteriorly for temporal bone removal.

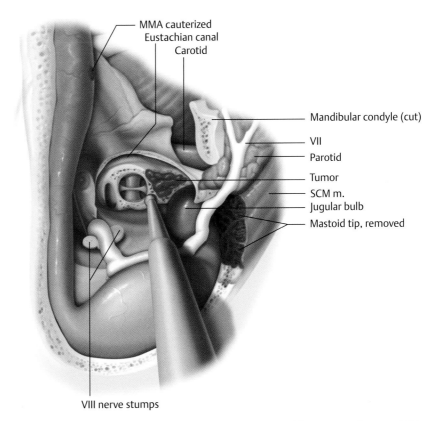

MMA cauterized
Eustachian canal
Carotid

Mandibular condyle (cut)
VII
Parotid
Tumor
SCM m.
Jugular bulb
Mastoid tip, removed

VIII nerve stumps

Fig. 13.11   Removal of the cochlea and the tumor. MMA, middle meningeal artery; SCM, sternocleidomastoid.

teum. If the tumor involves the protympanum, the mandibular condyle may be removed en bloc with the specimen, or an infratemporal fossa dissection may be performed (see below). Finally, the remaining cochlea and tumor are removed (**Fig. 13.11**). The eustachian tube is obliterated with bone wax, oxidized cellulose, and/or muscle. The cartilaginous component of the eustachian tube may be oversewn in addition to packing.

Extensions of the Subtotal Temporal Bone Resection

Further piecemeal removal of the temporal bone may be required to ensure total gross tumor removal and negative histologic margins.

Jugular Foramen

The neck is explored prior to bony dissection, and the internal jugular vein and cranial nerves IX through XII are identified and traced superiorly to the skull base. After bony dissection is completed and the tumor is debulked to a minimal portion attached to the jugular bulb/foramen, the internal jugular vein is doubly ligated with silk ties in the neck. Proximal control of the sigmoid sinus is achieved using oxidized cellulose packing extraluminally, underneath the remaining bony covering of sigmoid sinus. Extraluminal packing may also occlude the vein of Labbé; this event must be avoided as it may cause severe temporal lobe edema and venous infarction. If concomitant dural resection is anticipated, the sigmoid sinus is doubly ligated using a curved aneurysm needle just distal to the superior petrosal sinus. The involved,

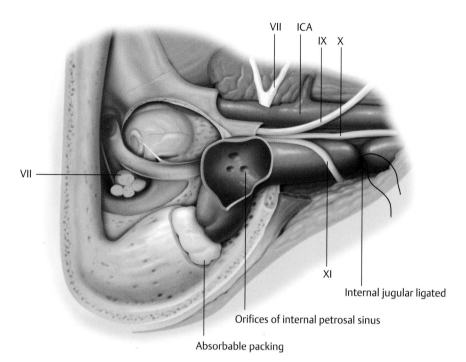

Fig. 13.12   Jugular bulb removal. ICA, internal carotid artery.

lateral venous wall of the sigmoid and jugular bulb is incised and removed. Brisk bleeding is to be expected from multiple areas along the medial wall of the jugular bulb from the inferior petrosal sinus. This bleeding is controlled with gentle pressure applied to Surgicel and with patience. If the tumor does not involve the medial jugular foramen and the lower cranial nerves are to be spared, care is taken not to traumatize these nerves with compression in an attempt to achieve hemostasis (**Fig. 13.12**).

If the tumor involves the medial aspect of the jugular foramen, the medial wall or the jugular bulb may be resected along with the contents of the pars nervosa. The ends of the lower cranial nerves may also be sent to the pathology laboratory for frozen section. The distal ends of the nerves may be followed into the neck until free of disease, as they are already exposed. The proximal ends of the nerves may be further followed into the posterior fossa until clear of disease. Further removal of bone medial to the jugular foramen may then be performed, if necessary.

If the lower cranial nerves are resected, rehabilitative measures to compensate for dysphagia and pulmonary aspiration may be performed. Options include tracheostomy and gastrostomy placement and/or medialization thyroplasty and arytenoid adduction.

Dural Resection

The temporal or posterior fossa dura may also be resected if involved with tumor, but this measure may or may not improve 5-year survival. A neurosurgical colleague is enlisted to aid in dural resection and closure. In the case of posterior fossa dural involvement, an incision may be made presigmoid and the involved dura removed with the cerebellum retracted posteromedially. For temporal lobe dural involvement, the incision is made superior and lateral to the area in question and the involved dura removed with the temporal lobe retracted superiorly. Dural closure may be achieved with fascia or a commercially available dural substitute such as Duragen or AlloDerm. Postoperative lumbar drainage is used to help decrease the risk of CSF leak from the dural resection.

Infratemporal Fossa

There may be gross tumor extension beyond the protympanum into the eustachian tube or anteriorly through the EAC wall into the infratemporal fossa. If this is the case, a total or radical parotidectomy is performed depending on the extent of facial nerve involvement with tumor. The skin incision is extended anteriorly to expose the entire temporalis muscle. The frontal branch of the facial nerve will have been identified through parotidectomy, or it will have been sacrificed. The zygomatic arch is approached in the plane of the temporal fat pad, just deep to the superficial layer of the temporalis fascia. The periosteum of the zygomatic arch is carefully dissected off of it along the entire length of the arch. The masseter muscle should also be released from its attachment to the zygoma. Osteotomies are made posteriorly at the zygomatic root and anteriorly near the malar eminence; the zygomatic arch is saved in physiologic solution. The temporalis muscle is sharply freed from its superior and posterior attachments and dissected bluntly off the underlying temporal squama, pedicled on the coronoid process of the mandible.

The mandibular condyle is subsequently resected. The articular disk and soft tissues of the temporomandibular joint are removed. With the zygomatic arch removed and temporalis muscle reflected inferiorly, the inferior surface of the skull base may be explored medially in a subperiosteal plane exposing the lateral pterygoid plate, V3, and the middle meningeal artery. The middle meningeal artery is doubly clipped or cauterized with a bipolar. The pterygoid muscles may be resected along with any gross tumor of the infratemporal fossa. Attempts to preserve the internal maxillary artery should be made, although this is not always possible. The reliability of the temporalis muscle as a reconstructive flap depends on the integrity of this artery and its collaterals. The vertical portion of the carotid artery should have been previously identified at its entry into the skull base, as should the cartilaginous eustachian tube, which can be further resected anteriorly to achieve negative tumor margin. More inferior exposure of the infratemporal fossa may be achieved if the styloid and all of its muscular and ligamentous attachments are removed. Care must be taken in doing this, as the internal carotid artery is just deep to these structures.

The temporal craniotomy from the translabyrinthine dissection can then be extended anteriorly and superiorly, exposing the temporal lobe dura along its lateral aspect. The temporal lobe may be elevated from the floor of the middle cranial fossa to the petrous ridge (bony side) and the superior petrosal sinus (dural side) medially, exposing the greater superficial petrosal nerve, and the intracranial side of V3 and the middle meningeal artery, which may be ligated again here. This approach allows excellent exposure above and below the floor of the middle cranial vault for further resection to achieve negative bony margins medially.

Total Temporal Bone Resection: Indications

Total temporal bone resection simply extends the subtotal resection beyond the internal carotid artery to include the anterior petrous apex. Resecting the ICA carries the inherent risk of devastating cerebral ischemia and infarction. The survival benefit of fully resecting the petrous apex in patients with advanced temporal bone carcinoma is often brought into question.

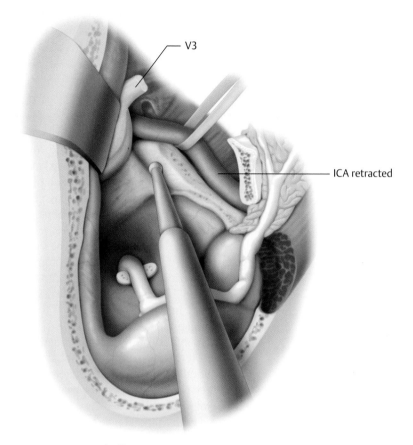

Fig. 13.13   Removal of bone in petrous apex. ICA, internal carotid artery.

Total Temporal Bone Resection: Procedure

A subtotal temporal bone resection has been performed. A vessel loop is placed around the infratemporal ICA for "control." The intrapetrous carotid is subsequently further exposed with diamond burs. The lateral aspect of the carotid is removed to the level of the foramen ovale and the distal carotid is mobilized from its canal. The remaining petrous apex can then be drilled away (**Fig. 13.13**).

Subtotal or Total Temporal Bone Resection: Reconstruction

As a subtotal or total temporal bone resection leads to exposure or opening of dural surfaces and transgression of the otic capsule, obliteration of the dead spaces and watertight closure is a necessity. The eustachian tube is obliterated with packing and/or oversewing of the distal end. Dural defects may be reconstructed with autologous or commercially available substitutes. In the case of a pure subtotal temporal bone resection, the soft tissue defect can be filled with temporalis muscle if its blood supply has not been compromised. For larger defects, a pedicled or free flap may be required. The closure is performed in multiple, staggered layers with 2-0 and 3-0 Vicryl sutures to decrease the risk of CSF leakage. The skin is closed in a watertight fashion using a running, locked 3-0 nylon or Prolene suture. A vascularized flap may include skin to replace skin removed with the specimen. If this is not the case, a skin graft may be required and a potential route of egress for CSF will result. To prevent a leak from occurring, the edges around the graft recipient site are meticulously tacked down with inverted, interrupted 3-0 Vicryl sutures to separate the actual graft bed from the deeper portions of the wound. A skin graft is then placed in the usual fashion with a bolster.

Cranial nerve reconstruction can also be performed at the time of resection, provided the margins are negative. For facial nerve defects of less than 6 cm, a greater auricular nerve graft can be used. One should bear in mind that this nerve itself may be involved with tumor, and it warrants histologic inspection if auricular numbness is a preoperative symptom. If greater length is required, a sural nerve graft may be harvested.

If facial nerve grafting is not possible or not attempted in the face of malignant involvement of the nerve, reconstitution of some facial nerve function may be obtained through a hypoglossal-facial anastomosis. The next options in order of decreasing desirability include dynamic or static slings. The patient's ability to close the ipsilateral eye may be facilitated with an upper lid gold weight or palpebral spring implantation.

Prior to complete wound closure, a Penrose drain is placed in patients with transgression of the CSF space; otherwise, a suction drain may be employed. A mastoid dressing is placed in patients who undergo lateral temporal bone resection and is left in place overnight. For those patients undergoing subtotal or total temporal bone resection, the choice of pressure dressing placement and duration is a balance between the decreasing risk of CSF leakage and the compromise of reconstructive flaps. Intraoperative lumbar drainage is continued postoperatively for 3 to 5 days, and then clamped. If no evidence of leak is noted with the drain clamped for 24 hours, it is removed.

◆ Complications and Adverse Events

Adverse perioperative events are more likely with increasing extent of tumor and resection and previous radiation therapy. The most serious consequences occur with subtotal and total temporal bone resections, as lateral temporal bone resection does not involve intracranial dissection. The most worrisome intraoperative event is bleeding from the ICA. Preoperative imaging should prepare the surgeon for dissection near, or sacrifice of, the ICA. Intraoperatively, proximal control of the vessel should be performed in the neck prior to manipulation along its infratemporal fossa and petrous segments. A damaged ICA can be repaired primarily, grafted, or possibly bypassed if collateral blood flow is questionable. In any situation where the ICA has been damaged, the patient should be monitored postoperatively for cerebral ischemia in an intensive care setting, preferably by an intensivist who is experienced in treating acute neurosurgical patients.

Neurologic events may also occur with damage or resection of the dural venous sinuses. Even with good contralateral venous outflow, the process of sacrificing the sigmoid sinus and jugular bulb may lead to inadvertent compromise of the vein of Labbé at its insertion into the lateral sinus. This compromise may lead to venous infarction or edema of the ipsilateral temporal lobe and cause speech abnormalities, if the dominant temporal lobe is affected, or seizures. Being aware of this possibility and packing the lateral sinus anterior to the vein of Labbé is the best way to prevent this result. Treatment of this event, should it occur, includes fluid management and anticonvulsant therapy. Long-term speech deficits are treated with speech therapy.

In the postoperative setting, an acute intracranial hemorrhage may occur. These patients may present with altered sensorium, acute anisocoria, hemiparesis, and aphasia. Depending on the rapidity and nature of the symptoms and proximity to the operating room, the patient may be rushed back to the operating room for wound exploration, evacuation of blood clot, and control of bleeding vessels. If the clinical scenario is less clear, the patient may undergo emergent head CT scanning with possible operative intervention if a bleed is noted.

Another postoperative complication that may occur is wound breakdown with exposure of vital structures underneath. This complication is more likely to occur in the setting of prior radiation therapy to the operative site. If great vessels or dura will potentially be exposed with a failing reconstruction, wound debridement and an alternative reconstruction must urgently be performed. Wound infection is a rare event, but may increase the risk of CSF infection and meningitis and must be dealt with accordingly with IV antibiotics and possible wound debridement.

Intracranial infections include meningitis and abscess. Patients with fever, worsening headache, neck rigidity, and altered cognition should initially receive intravenous antibiotics and a contrasted head CT followed by an MRI if abscess is suspected. We prefer vancomycin and ceftazidime for their CSF penetration and combined broad spectrum of coverage. A lumbar puncture is performed and the CSF examined and cultured. Surgical drainage is indicated for treatment of intracranial abscess with IV antibiotics; bacterial meningitis is treated with IV antibiotics and possibly steroids. The length of antibiotic use varies depending on the findings at workup and at repeat CSF examination(s).

Cerebrospinal fluid leak can occur through the eustachian tube and nose or through the wound itself. The most devastating consequence of a CSF fistula is seeding of bacteria to the subarachnoid space and ensuing meningitis. The best way to avoid these complications is by prevention through meticulous eustachian tube packing, watertight wound closure, and lumbar drainage if a large dural defect results from the resection. In those cases where a leak occurs, a patient may benefit from initiation or continuation of lumbar drainage for 3 to 5 days. The patient is placed on bed rest, and lumbar drain is begun at 6 mL/h and titrated upward until a mild spinal headache is experienced. After 3 to 5 days, the drain is clamped for 24 hours and removed if the leakage ceases. For wound leaks, a pressure dressing and wound overclosure with 0-nylon or 0-silk may be performed. If these conservative measures fail at resolving CSF leakage, then the patient is brought back to the operating room for wound exploration and repair of the fistula.

◆ Conclusion

Temporal bone removal remains the main therapy for malignancies of the temporal bone. The extent of dissection is determined by the tumor's temporal bone involvement. This usually requires either a lateral temporal bone resection, which includes external ear canal and tympanic membrane, or a total temporal bone resection that may require dural resection or be extradural. Postoperative radiation therapy is required in many cases, and reconstruction with vascularized flaps is required to prevent subsequent CSF leak after radiation therapy.

Suggested Readings
Arriaga M, Curtin H, Takahashi H, Hirsch BE, Kamerer DB. Staging proposal for external auditory meatus carcinoma based on preoperative clinical examination and computed tomography findings. Ann Otol Rhinol Laryngol 1990;99(9 Pt 1):714–721

Graham MD, Sataloff RT, Kemink JL, Wolf GT, McGillicuddy JE. Total en bloc resection of the temporal bone and carotid artery for malignant tumors of the ear and temporal bone. Laryngoscope 1984; 94:528–533

Kinney SE. Squamous cell carcinoma of the external auditory canal. Am J Otol 1989;10:111–116

Lewis JS, Page R. Radical surgery for malignant tumors of the ear. Arch Otolaryngol 1966;83:114–119

Moffat DA, Wagstaff SA, Hardy DG. The outcome of radical surgery and postoperative radiotherapy for squamous carcinoma of the temporal bone. Laryngoscope 2005;115:341–347

Moody SA, Hirsch BE, Myers EN. Squamous cell carcinoma of the external auditory canal: an evaluation of a staging system. Am J Otol 2000;21:582–588

Prasad S, Janecka IP. Efficacy of surgical treatments for squamous cell carcinoma of the temporal bone: a literature review. Otolaryngol Head Neck Surg 1994;110:270–280

14

Microvascular Cranial Nerve Decompression

Marc S. Schwartz and Derald E. Brackmann

The scope of lateral skull base surgery includes surgical treatment of the group of disorders known as microvascular compression syndromes. The most common of these, and the first attributed to the pathology of microvascular compression, is trigeminal neuralgia. Trigeminal neuralgia is marked by unilateral, severe, lancinating facial pain elicited by triggering and (at least partially) relieved by carbamazepine. Each of the other microvascular compression syndromes is defined by a characteristic clinical presentation and is associated with a specific cranial nerve. These are trigeminal neuralgia (trigeminal nerve), hemifacial spasm (facial nerve), geniculate neuralgia (nervus intermedius), severe positional vertigo (vestibular nerve), and glossopharyngeal neuralgia (glossopharyngeal nerve). An understanding of the clinical presentation of each of these disorders is critical to successful treatment.

Also critical to the treatment of these patients is an understanding that treatment is always done for quality-of-life reasons. None of these disorders is directly life-threatening, and invasive treatment should be undertaken only after all medical options have been exhausted and only if symptomatology is severe. On the other hand, patients can be assured that, in proper hands, these disorders can safely and effectively be treated with surgery if it becomes necessary.

Microvascular decompression (MVD) of each of these nerves is performed via retrosigmoid craniotomy. The goal is isolation of the affected cranial nerve from any compressing vascular structures. Although magnetic resonance imaging (MRI) is useful in confirming the presence of microvascular compression, it should be remembered that each vascular compression syndrome is a clinical diagnosis. We obtain a preoperative MRI for every patient. The main reason to obtain an MRI is to exclude the possibility of tumor or other compressive lesion such as arachnoid cyst and to ensure that there is no intrinsic brain abnormality, such as brainstem infarct or multiple sclerosis plaque, which would contraindicate microvascular decompression. MR sequences such as constructive interference in steady state (CISS) and fast imaging employing steady state acquisition (FIESTA) show the anatomy of the cranial nerves with very good detail. However, the surgeon should not be dissuaded from performing MVD in the absence of MR evidence of microvascular compression if there is a compelling clinical picture.

◆ Surgical Technique

Microvascular decompression is performed via a retrosigmoid craniotomy. We utilize continuous facial nerve and auditory brainstem response monitoring for all cases. The patient is positioned supine on the operating table and is carefully secured to allow rotation of the table. The table may be flexed slightly to create a "lounge" position, which lowers the shoulder in relation to the operative line-of-sight. A Mayfield headholder is used with the head rotated 45 to 60 degrees contralaterally. The neck is flexed slightly, although care is taken with positioning to avoid overrotation and interference with venous return in the neck. For trigeminal nerve decompression, the vertex is dropped to allow for less hindered access below the tentorium. For decompression of the other nerves, a relatively neutral position can be utilized in this access. The surgeon sits behind the patient's head.

As the craniotomy must be oriented to the transverse-sigmoid junction, an appreciation of the courses of these structures is critical. The transverse sinus runs at the level of the zygomatic arch (the Frankfurt line), and the sigmoid sinus is located at the posterior edge of the mastoid. Of course, there is significant individual variation. A curved incision is utilized with its apex approximately three fingerbreadths behind the ear. The scalp is elevated forward toward the mastoid, and an inverted L-shaped incision is made in the periosteum with limbs over the mastoid process and the inferior temporal line. The suboccipital muscles are elevated in a separate flap inferiorly and medially. We prefer this overlapping flap technique rather than a smaller linear incision to prevent postoperative cerebrospinal fluid (CSF) leak.

A small craniotomy is performed in the retrosigmoid area using cutting and diamond burs. This craniotomy must include exposure of the posterior edge of the sigmoid sinus and the inferior edge of the transverse sinus. Proper placement is facilitated by entry into the mastoid air cells, via which the inner table over the sigmoid sinus can be directly visualized. It is often necessary to drill away a significant amount of bone to properly orient the bone flap and to expose and control any emissary veins. Being left with a tiny bone flap, or performing a craniectomy, is preferable to lacerating the sinus or to having an improperly positioned bony opening. We aim for a craniotomy approximately 2.5 cm along the sigmoid sinus and 2 cm along the transvers sinus. After removal of bone, any exposed mastoid air cells are occluded with bone wax.

Opening of the dura must be performed with great care. The dura is nicked with a scalpel and CSF is drained from over the cerebellar hemisphere. If no CSF is obtained, the patient may be placed in the reverse Trendelenburg position. Also, the attainment of adequate diuresis and hyperventilation should be confirmed with the anesthesiologist. An inferior dural opening is performed, extending to the lower edge of the exposed sigmoid sinus. After a cottonoid is advanced over the cerebellum adjacent to the inferior aspect of the petrous bone, the cerebellum is gently retracted using a microsucker. The working space in this area can be very narrow, and great care is taken to advance to the arachnoid overlying the cisterna magna. The cistern is opened using a sharp micro–nerve hook, and with the egress of CSF, brain relaxation is achieved. The dural opening is completed only after the brain is relaxed to prevent herniation. Care is taken to ensure that the opening is brought to the edge of the sigmoid sinus, as every extra millimeter of exposure paralleling the sigmoid is critical.

For microvascular decompression of all nerves, wide arachnoid dissection is critical. It is important not only for direct exposure of the involved nerve, but also for mobilization of the cerebellar hemisphere. With adequate dissection, only minimal cerebellar retraction, if any, is necessary to visualize both nerves and the brainstem surface. For trigeminal nerve decompression, sacrifice of one or more bridging petrosal veins may be required. For other nerves, this is generally unnecessary. Small arteries bridging to the petrous bone may be sacrificed only if they are laterally placed and clearly distant from the neural foramina. These are usually small loops that become adherent to the dura and supply blood to the lateral aspects of the cerebellum. If retraction is needed, a narrow retractor blade with a bluntly hooked end is ideal. Using this type of retractor, cerebellar hemisphere, flocculus, or even choroids plexus can be gently raised instead of being pushed, thus maximizing exposure while minimizing pressure on the cerebellum and traction on the cranial nerves.

Decompression is performed using Teflon felt (Bard PV, Inc., Tempe, AZ), which is teased to create small, fluffy pieces. Individual teased pieces are rolled to form pledgets of various sizes, approximating the size and shape of grains of rice. Pledgets are not used without proper hydration. Dissection and pledget insertion is performed with minimal retraction, using preferably only a manually held suction, and, if necessary, self-retaining retractors. If any changes occur with auditory brainstem response (ABR) monitoring, retraction is immediately released.

After completion of the MVD, closure is performed. If the patient has been placed in the reverse Trendelenburg position, the head is lowered to a neutral position. The cranial nerves are reinspected after irrigation to ensure that they remain well decompressed. We make no attempt to close the dura in a watertight manner. Instead, the dura is tacked together and overlaid with an onlay collagenous matrix graft. Cranioplasty is always performed, as previously described for the retrosigmoid route, and the wound is closed in layers.

We utilize the operating microscope as the primary aid to visualization for MVDs. Endoscopic assistance, however, is very beneficial as an adjunct. The chief advantages of the endoscopic viewpoint are the ability to view at an angle and a wider field of view. These advantages are of particular utility for MVD. The major disadvantage is visual acuity, which is, at this point, clearly inferior to the microscope. In contrast to tumor dissection, however, modern endoscopes and video equipment are in practice generally adequate for these procedures. Before attempting any dissection under endoscopic guidance, the surgeon should become comfortable simply observing the operative field using first a 0-degree endoscope and then a 30-degree angled endoscope. Only after gaining full comfort with these endoscopes should the surgeon begin to utilize a fixed endoscope holder and then carry out any dissection (bimanually). We would not recommend the use of endoscopes angled greater than 30 degrees, as they are generally more awkward to advance in the cerebellopontine angle.

Trigeminal Nerve

For microvascular decompression of the trigeminal nerve, it is useful to tilt the vertex downward to facilitate exposure directly along the tentorium. Although the eventual goal is superior, initial dissection to open the basal cisterns is performed inferiorly along the petrous ridge. An arachnoid opening is performed over the lower cranial nerves and the cranial nerve VII–VIII complex prior to advancing toward the trigeminal nerve. All bridging petrosal veins are coagulated and divided, and the superior portion of the cerebellar hemisphere is gently retracted.

It is necessary to visualize the entire length of the trigeminal nerve from the pons to the entrance to Meckel's cave (**Fig. 14.1**). The motor branch is seen just medial to the main trunk of the nerve. Microvascular compression can be the result of either arterial or venous structures, and there are often multiple vessels seen. The nerve must be isolated from all vascular structures. When compression is the result of veins only, an arterial loop can typically be seen compressing the vein, which transmits arterial pulsations to the nerve.

All arterial loops are carefully dissected away from the nerve using microinstruments. Microspatulas and very fine but blunt micro–nerve hooks are useful. Veins can be coagulated and divided with care. It is critical to be certain that there is no compression from medial or superior to the nerve, as these orientations will be less obvious than the opposing directions. Special attention must be paid to the most proximal portion of the nerve near the brainstem, and the adjacent root entry zone must be isolated from vascular compression as well (**Fig. 14.2**).

The area of the nerve more distal in the cistern, while most easily visualized, is also the most difficult to adequately decompress. Although arterial loops in this region can be dissected free of the nerve, veins must be handled delicately. It is occasionally impossible to safely separate veins from the nerve in this region. These veins can be

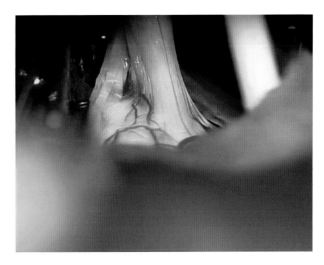

Fig. 14.1 Microsurgical exposure of the trigeminal nerve for MVD (right side). The nerve must be visualized over its entire length, including the root entry zone. The motor branch is seen superoanterior to the main sensory nerve.

coagulated and divided well away from the nerve. This will effectively devitalize the veins as they pass the nerve. Care must be taken to ensure not only that the nerve is isolated from any arterial loops but also that any venous fragments are as well.

Facial Nerve

Decompression of the facial nerve is particularly difficult due to its proximity to the vestibulocochlear nerve, which is particularly sensitive to trauma, including stretch. Wide arachnoid dissection is necessary to visualize the entire length of the facial nerve. Opening is performed over the lower cranial nerves and the cranial nerve VII–VIII complex. It is critical to visualize the space between these two nerve bundles all the way to the brainstem surface. The facial nerve takes a curving course, and its

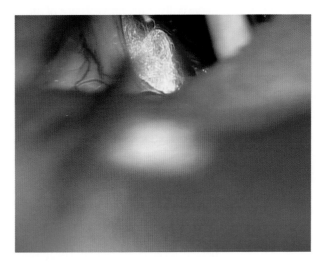

Fig. 14.2 Microsurgical view of decompression of the root entry zone of the trigeminal nerve. Teased Teflon felt is utilized.

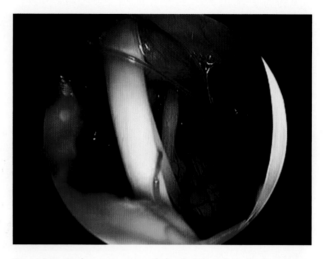

Fig. 14.3 Endoscopic view of the facial and vestibulocochlear nerves. The facial nerve runs anteriorly and curves inferiorly to reach its root entry zone. The facial nerve root entry zone lies anteriorly in the space between the facial and glossopharyngeal nerves and must be meticulously explored.

proximal segment extends along the brainstem inferiorly, anterior to the lower cranial nerves (**Fig. 14.3**). A good guide is the choroid plexus. The choroid must be well visualized and protected with a micro-cottonoid as it is gently retracted to gain access to the region anterior to it.

Microvascular compression causing hemifacial spasm is usually caused by an arterial loop. Loops of anterior inferior cerebellar artery (AICA) branches may be located along the course of the facial nerve in the cistern. Often, a loop will extend through the space between the facial nerve and the vestibulocochlear nerve. It is important to probe the space between any such vessel and the facial nerve all the way to the porus. A branch of this vessel invariably runs into the internal auditory canal (IAC), supplying the inner ear. Injury to this branch will result in disruption of vestibulocochlear function. Exploration of the brainstem surface at the root entry zone of the facial nerve is also imperative. Loops of the AICA or posterior inferior cerebellar artery (PICA) may be in contact with the facial nerve or its root entry zone. If this area is neglected, results will be poor.

As stated above, special care is necessary with facial nerve microvascular decompression to avoid injury to the vestibulocochlear nerve. ABRs are carefully monitored. If any changes occur, dissection is ceased and retraction is relaxed until these changes revert. Total loss of ABR waveform predicts loss of cochlear and vestibular function. If dissection is otherwise meticulous, this occurrence is likely due to vascular injury. For this reason, sacrifice of even very small arteries is avoided.

Nervus Intermedius

The nervus intermedius runs along the superior edge of the cranial nerve VII–VIII complex, often in a groove created by these two larger nerves. Its visualization may be aided with a 30-degree angled endoscope. If involvement of this nerve is suspected, it can be sectioned. The nervus intermedius is carefully isolated, often blindly, using a micro–nerve hook and divided using a fine microscissors. We have not performed nervus intermedius section as an isolated procedure. Rather, it has been performed in cases with atypical features, with predominant ear neuralgia-type pain, in conjunction with microvascular decompression of the trigeminal and/or glossopharyngeal nerves.

Vestibular Nerve

Within the confines of the IAC, the vestibulocochlear nerve divides into its three components: the superior and inferior vestibular nerves and the cochlear nerve. In its cisternal portion, the vestibulocochlear is a single entity, without well-defined divisions. Vestibular fibers run along the superior half of the nerve. There may be a small vessel running along the posterior aspect nerve demarcating the line between the vestibular and cochlear portions, but this is inconsistent.

Severe positional vertigo, or motion intolerance, is thought to be potentially due to microvascular compression of the vestibular fibers in the cerebellopontine angle cistern or at the root entry zone. A loop of the AICA is often found in this location and in contact with the nerve. Veins running along the brainstem surface are often found as well.

Because of the lack of clear objective criteria for decompression of the vestibular portion of the vestibulocochlear nerve, we carry out a less aggressive microvascular decompression. The fact that any definitively lateralizing symptoms, signs, or diagnostic tests for this disorder are lacking also argues for a less aggressive approach. In the performance of MVD for this nerve, brain retraction is shunned, and any changes in ABR monitoring during nerve dissection are regarded with the utmost seriousness.

Decompression of cranial nerve VIII is not carried into the IAC. No drilling is done, and the IAC components are not exposed. Frequently, an arterial loop runs along the nerve toward the porus. This loop typically gives rise to a branch that enters the IAC to supply the inner ear structures. Special care is taken to avoid disruption of this branch, even if this makes adequate decompression difficult or impossible.

The entire cranial nerve VIII is decompressed, including both the vestibular and the cochlear portions. Visualization of vessels along the medialmost portion of the nerves is facilitated by sharp dissection of the flocculus from the nerve. Veins on the brainstem surface at the root entry zone represent a particular challenge. They cannot be dissected free and must be coagulated and divided. Coagulation is performed at a location distant from any neural structures to avoid thermal or electrical damage.

Glossopharyngeal Nerve

Access to the region of the glossopharyngeal nerve is straightforward. After CSF is released from the cisterna magna, arachnoid is opened over the lower cranial nerves and superiorly to the cerebellopontine angle. Microvascular compression is most commonly the result of a loop of the PICA, which can be separated from the lower cranial nerves in a straightforward fashion. A sizable PICA loop may run posterior to the glossopharyngeal nerve and may indent the brainstem in the region of the lateral recess. Decompression of such a vessel is a routine matter, although all small branches must be preserved, and the choroids plexus must be protected.

In rare cases, microvascular compression may result from a tortuous vertebral artery. This large vessel runs anteromedial to the lower cranial nerves, and its manipulation may be problematic. The vertebral artery is handled gently, and adequate decompression requires manipulation of the nerve fibers themselves. As Teflon pledgets are inserted, nerve fibers are retracted away from the vessel rather than the reverse. Creation of a suture sling to hold nerve fibers away from the vessel, or the reverse, has been described, but we have not utilized this technique.

In cases where adequate decompression of the glossopharyngeal nerve from an offending vertebral artery is difficult, either total or partial sectioning of the glossopharyngeal nerve can be considered. However, we would not typically recommend nerve section with the first procedure. In difficult cases, microvascular decompression is performed as best as possible with the first procedure. If ineffective, the patient is reexplored with the intension of performing glossopharyngeal nerve section.

◆ Technical Pearls

- Diagnosis of microvascular compression syndromes is made primarily on the basis of clinical symptoms rather than radiographic findings.
- Extensive arachnoid dissection from trigeminal to lower cranial nerves is necessary for MVD of any nerve.
- Nerves must be visualized entirely, from root entry zone to foramina.
- Nerves (and root entry zones) must be isolated from all vessels, including arteries and veins.

◆ Conclusion

For appropriately selected patients, microvascular decompression can be performed routinely for a variety of problems that may severely impact the patient's quality of life. Exploration of entire nerves, with particular attention to root entry zones, is crucial to success. Both surgical microscope and endoscope are useful adjuncts to these procedures.

Suggested Readings

Barker FG II, Jannetta PJ, Bissonette DJ, Shields PT, Larkins MV, Jho HD. Microvascular decompression for hemifacial spasm. J Neurosurg 1995;82:201–210

Lovely TJ, Jannetta PJ. Microvascular decompression for trigeminal neuralgia. Surgical technique and long-term results. Neurosurg Clin N Am 1997;8:11–29 Review

Lovely TJ, Jannetta PJ. Surgical management of geniculate neuralgia. Am J Otol 1997;18:512–517

McLaughlin MR, Jannetta PJ, Clyde BL, Subach BR, Comey CH, Resnick DK. Microvascular decompression of cranial nerves: lessons learned after 4400 operations. J Neurosurg 1999;90:1–8

Møller MB, Møller AR, Jannetta PJ, Jho HD, Sekhar LN. Microvascular decompression of the eighth nerve in patients with disabling positional vertigo: selection criteria and operative results in 207 patients. Acta Neurochir (Wien) 1993;125:75–82

Resnick DK, Jannetta PJ, Bissonnette D, Jho HD, Lanzino G. Microvascular decompression for glossopharyngeal neuralgia. Neurosurgery 1995;36:64–68, discussion 68–69

15

Complications of Neurotologic Surgery

John W. House and Robert D. Cullen

The treatment of vestibular schwannomas (VSs) and other skull base lesions has evolved quite remarkably since the first surgery for VS was described by Ballance in 1895. Whereas the reduction in mortality was the focus of surgical advancement in the first half of the 20th century, the reduction in morbidity associated with cranial neuropathies has been the goal since that time. This has largely been accomplished with the introduction of the microscope to neurotology, intraoperative cranial nerve monitoring, and advances in neuroanesthesia.

Despite the current low incidence of complications of neurotologic surgery, an understanding of the pathogenesis, predisposing contributing factors, and management of these complications is critical.

◆ Preoperative Workup

Prevention of complications begins with a careful preoperative evaluation of the patient. A careful neurotologic examination will reveal preexisting neurologic deficits such as facial weakness or numbness, signs of cerebellar compression, and hydrocephalus. Preoperative imaging aids in confirming not only the tumor type and size, but also the relationship of the tumor to surrounding neurovascular structures. Tumor size and proximity to critical structures is directly related to anticipated complications and cranial nerve deficits.

An appropriate medical evaluation of the patient is also mandatory. Medical comorbidities should be identified and controlled as well as possible prior to subjecting the patient to a neurotologic procedure. At our institution, we include in the health care team an internist experienced with the care of the neurotologic patient. This expertise has greatly augmented the perioperative care of our patients.

◆ Complications

Cerebrospinal Fluid Leak

Cerebrospinal fluid (CSF) leak is one of the most common complication of acoustic neuroma surgery, with a reported incidence of 2 to 30%. This problem persists despite advancement in acoustic tumor surgical techniques, and contributes to prolonged hospital stays and postoperative meningitis. Our current rate of CSF leak at the House Clinic is 4.3%, which compares favorably with the 9.4% incidence published in the past. Only one third of patients who experience a postoperative CSF leak require an additional procedure for control of the leak. The remaining patients are managed conservatively. We attribute this low incidence to our current intraoperative closure practice, as outlined below.

The diagnosis of CSF leak is usually very straightforward in the patient who has recently undergone skull base surgery. CSF leakage is usually manifested as either rhinorrhea or leakage through the surgical wound. Rarely, CSF otorrhea will occur. The evaluation of idiopathic CSF leak is beyond the scope of this chapter and will not be discussed further. Special tests to confirm the diagnosis of postoperative CSF leak are rarely required.

In any surgical approach to acoustic neuroma, the pneumatized air cell system of the temporal bone is entered, and a potential communication between the temporal bone and the subarachnoid space can persist, resulting in leakage of CSF through the skin incision or the eustachian tube (presenting as rhinorrhea). Despite differences in technique, no significant difference in the rate of CSF leaks among the translabyrinthine, retrosigmoid, and middle fossa approaches to acoustic tumor surgery has been shown.

Closure of a translabyrinthine craniotomy involves obliteration of the partial dural defect with fat harvested from the lower abdomen. The fat is cut into strips and soaked in bacitracin. The dura is closed along the posterior fossa incision, and fat strips are tightly packed into the dural opening and the internal auditory canal (IAC), extending 2 cm into the cerebellopontine angle. Additional fat is packed in the mastoid defect. The incus is removed and the eustachian tube is filled with Surgicel mixed with bone wax, followed by muscle. The middle ear space is also obliterated with muscle. Alternatively, the incus may be left in place and the antrum packed with muscle. A titanium cranioplasty mesh is inserted over the mastoid cavity to better secure the fat grafts. Any air cells exposed during the procedure are sealed with bone wax. The wound is closed in layers and a pressure dressing is applied.

Following tumor removal in a retrosigmoid approach, we prefer to use bone wax to seal all exposed air cells. The petrosal defect created after opening of the IAC is packed with abdominal fat and secured with dural suture or fibrin glue. The wound is then closed in layers, and a compressive dressing is applied.

In a middle cranial fossa approach, all exposed air cells are waxed and obliterated with abdominal fat, and the IAC is filled with abdominal fat. Air cells or dehiscences in the floor of the middle cranial fossa are waxed or covered with fascia. Following release of retraction of the temporal lobe, any dural defects are repaired with suture or fat graft. The craniotomy bone flap is replaced, the wound closed, and a pressure dressing is applied.

Management of the patient with a postoperative CSF leak must be tailored to the hearing status of the patient, as well as the site of the fistula. A variety of options for treatment exist, ranging from conservative measures such as bed rest and lumbar drainage to surgical revision. Below is a logical algorithm used at the House Clinic for management of postoperative CSF leaks (**Fig. 15.1**).

Various protocols for conservative management of CSF leaks have been described. A recent meta-analysis of 25 studies concluded that for incisional leaks, conservative management, including wound resuturing, pressure dressings, bed rest, and head elevation, is indicated for the first 48 hours. Should this fail to control the leak, continuous lumbar drainage may be performed for 2 to 5 days. Surgical reexploration is indicated for persistent leaks. Cases of rhinorrhea do not respond well to conservative management, and thus are treated initially with 2 to 5 days of lumbar drainage, followed by surgical revision for recalcitrant leaks. We prefer early surgical intervention to prevent the development of meningitis seen with prolonged leaks.

Surgical management of recalcitrant CSF leaks first involves exploration of the craniotomy cavity. Abdominal fat used during the primary surgery is removed and repacked. Any air cell tracts that are discovered are sealed with bone wax and abdominal fat. In patients without serviceable hearing, the middle ear is also obliterated with abdominal fat, and the eustachian tube orifice is sealed with bone wax and a muscle

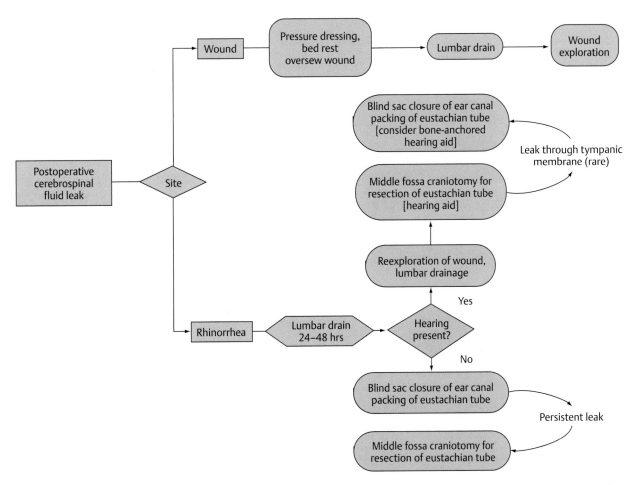

Fig. 15.1 House Clinic algorithm for the management of cerebrospinal fluid (CSF) leak after craniotomy. From Friedman RA, Cullen RD, Ulis J, Brackmann DE. Management of cerebrospinal fluid leaks after acoustic tumor removal. Neurosurgery 2007;61(3 Suppl): 35–39. Reprinted by permission.

graft (**Fig. 15.2**). The ear canal is closed in a blind-sac fashion. This is done so that the anterior bony annulus may be removed to expose the introitus of the eustachian tube. It is important to carefully examine all possible dural sources of CSF leakage as well as potential air cell routes to the eustachian tube. Revision surgery is nearly 100% effective in treating CSF rhinorrhea when a correctable defect is observed.

Occasionally, a patient does not have an observable defect and rhinorrhea will be recalcitrant to surgical treatment. In our experience, using a middle fossa approach to section and pack the eustachian tube has been effective in blocking the final common pathway for CSF flow (**Fig. 15.3**). This technique allows for a disruption of the communication to the middle ear without relying on eustachian tube packing materials that may potentially become porous or nonobstructive over time. In this procedure, a middle fossa craniotomy is performed. The epitympanum is opened and the tensor tympani muscle removed. The eustachian tube can then be followed through its bony course. Exposed air cells are sealed with bone wax. The cartilaginous eustachian tube is identified and divided, and a segmental portion removed. Both ends are cauterized, packed with cellulose and muscle, and occluded with bone wax. After careful examination for air cells, the bone flap from the craniotomy is secured with titanium miniplates. A layered closure is performed and a compressive dressing is applied. In all

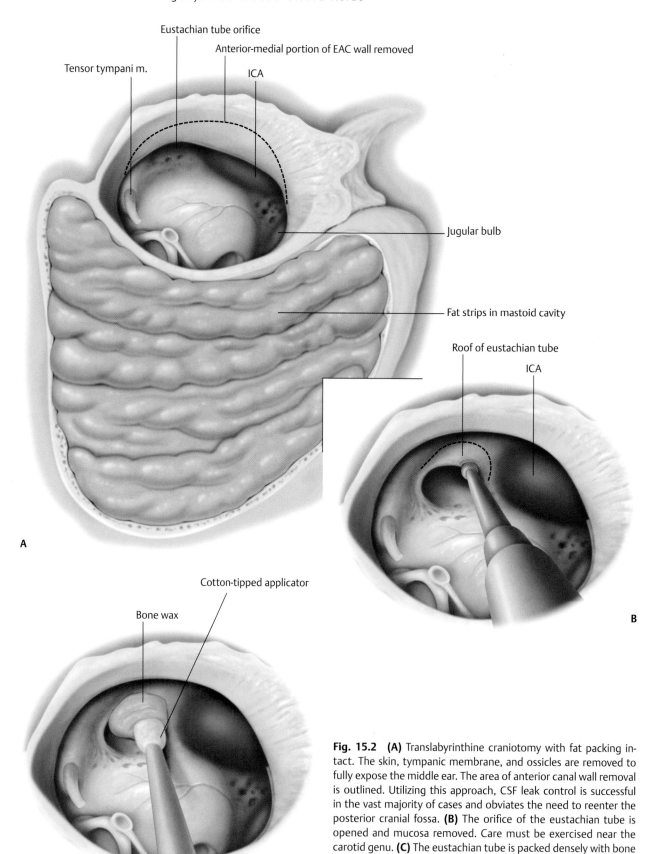

Tensor tympani m.

Eustachian tube orifice

Anterior-medial portion of EAC wall removed

ICA

Jugular bulb

Fat strips in mastoid cavity

Roof of eustachian tube

ICA

A

B

Cotton-tipped applicator

Bone wax

C

Fig. 15.2 **(A)** Translabyrinthine craniotomy with fat packing intact. The skin, tympanic membrane, and ossicles are removed to fully expose the middle ear. The area of anterior canal wall removal is outlined. Utilizing this approach, CSF leak control is successful in the vast majority of cases and obviates the need to reenter the posterior cranial fossa. **(B)** The orifice of the eustachian tube is opened and mucosa removed. Care must be exercised near the carotid genu. **(C)** The eustachian tube is packed densely with bone under direct vision. EAC, external auditory canal; ICA, internal carotid artery.

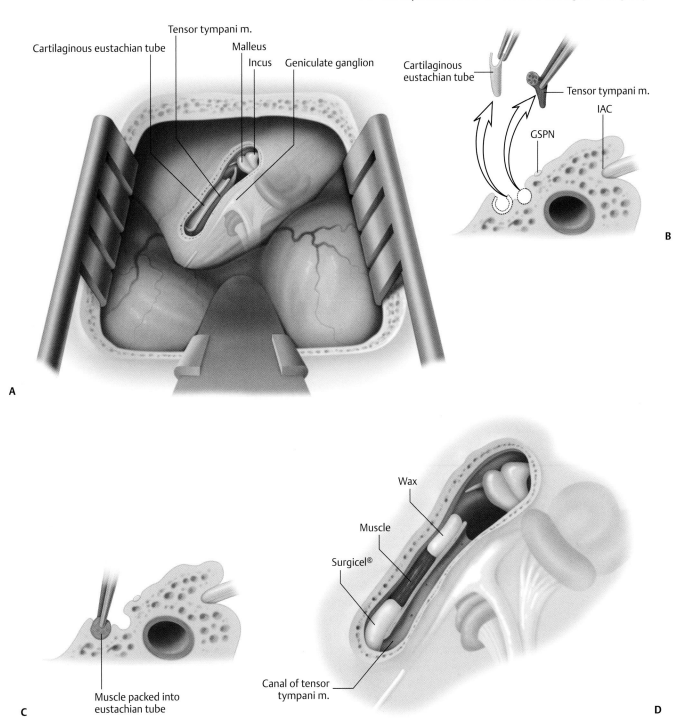

Fig. 15.3 **(A)** Middle cranial fossa exposure in a right temporal bone. The eustachian tube is identified from above in its full length. Care must be taken to avoid the adjacent petrous carotid artery. The roof of the semicanal for the tensor tympani is removed and the eustachian tube is identified inferiorly. **(B,C)** Coronal view of the eustachian tube and petrous carotid artery. Tensor tympani muscle is resected first, revealing the cartilaginous eustachian tube. The cartilaginous tube is resected and the distal end oversewn. **(D)** Completion of eustachian tube obliteration. GSPN, greater superficial petrosal nerve; IAC, internal auditory canal.

cases that this approach has been attempted, recalcitrant leak has resolved, and we therefore recommend it in difficult cases that fail a first surgical revision.

Infection

Wound infection and meningitis are uncommon complications due to the use of prophylactic antibiotics and meticulous surgical technique. All patients undergoing neurotologic surgery are administered antibiotics immediately prior to surgery and for the first postoperative day. As the majority of cases occur in clean surgical fields, infection rates are very low.

Meningitis usually occurs as a complication of a postoperative CSF leak. Bacteria gain access to the subarachnoid space via the surgical wound or, more commonly, the eustachian tube. The typical symptoms of headache, meningismus, and fever are usually present. However, these symptoms may be masked by the use of postoperative steroids. Lumbar puncture and culture are necessary to confirm the diagnosis and to select the appropriate antibiotic therapy. It is preferable to start empiric antibiotics after the lumbar puncture; however, there should be no significant delay in the administration of antibiotics. Early, aggressive therapy for meningitis helps to eliminate any long-term morbidity associated with meningitis.

Stroke

Cerebral ischemia may be the result of arterial or venous injury. Preoperative planning will include an evaluation of the vessels involved in the approach and removal of the tumor. If indicated, preoperative angiography with balloon occlusion of the internal carotid artery (ICA) may be performed. Xenon computed tomography (CT) perfusion studies are useful in predicting the sufficiency of collateral circulation; however, these studies are not infallible and will not account for possible retrograde thrombosis into the collateral circulation of a sacrificed ICA. It is therefore inadvisable to sacrifice the ICA for benign disease. In addition, given the poor prognosis of patients who require ICA sacrifice for malignant disease, there is a very limited role for this practice in modern skull base surgery.

The anterior inferior cerebellar artery (AICA) is at risk of injury in the microsurgical treatment of vestibular schwannoma. If injured in the proximal segment, patients will develop a lateral pontomedullary syndrome, characterized by ataxia, dysmetria, facial numbness and weakness, ipsilateral Horner's syndrome, and contralateral paresthesia of the body. Ipsilateral dysmetria is characteristic due to ischemia of the cerebellar outflow tracts through the superior cerebellar peduncle. Severe brainstem dysfunction may lead to prolonged hospitalization or death.

A distal AICA injury results in less severe sequelae. Dysarthria, dysmetria, ataxia, and dysdiadokinesia are common signs. Perhaps the earliest clue to an AICA injury after skull base surgery is abnormal ipsilateral saccades, which may differentiate the other symptoms of hearing loss, facial weakness, vertigo, and nausea from the effects of lateral skull base surgery. Supportive measures and physical and speech rehabilitation are provided in these cases. A good long-term recovery can be expected, with minimal sequelae after 1 year.

Venous complications may also occur. Sacrifice of the jugular bulb or sigmoid sinus may result in cerebral edema due to poor venous drainage of the brain. Extensive retraction of the temporal lobe in petroclival or extended middle fossa approaches may risk the compromise of the inferior anastomotic cerebral vein (vein of Labbé). The vein of Labbé drains into the transverse sinus a variable distance from the sigmoid sinus. If the superior anastomotic cerebral vein of Trolard is not patent or of small caliber, the vein of Labbé will provide the only veinous drainage of the entire ipsilateral cerebral hemisphere. Sacrifice of this vein would lead to massive infarction and often death.

Cerebral Edema

Cerebral edema may occur from the direct effects of brain retraction or the compromise of major draining veins. Extensive and prolonged retraction must be avoided and the posterior temporal veins, and veins of the posterior fossa should be preserved when possible. Diagnosis is made by recognizing a neurologic decline in the patient and confirmed by CT or magnetic resonance imaging (MRI) findings. Treatment is supportive, including fluid restriction, hyperventilation, steroids and the use of osmotic agents. Lumbar drainage, if used, should be discontinued. If excessive temporal lobe edema occurs, uncal herniation is possible, and should be treated with immediate surgical decompression.

Cranial Nerve Deficits

Facial nerve dysfunction, although once routine, has since declined with the modern use of microdissection and facial nerve monitoring. Anatomic preservation of the facial nerve is now standard, whereas long-term functional outcomes vary. Long-term facial function outcome is primarily dependent on the size of the tumor and the proximity to the facial nerve. If the facial nerve is transected, immediate grafting should be performed with a greater auricular nerve or sural nerve graft. House-Brackmann grade III or IV function can be expected with a primary interposition graft.

The care of the paralyzed face is of utmost importance, particularly with regard to the eye. If trigeminal dysfunction is also present, the anesthetic cornea is at significant risk of injury. Eyedrops and lubricants are instituted as well as other protective mechanisms. Taping of the eye, moisture chambers, and bandage contact lenses are all temporary measures of corneal protection. The consultation of an ophthalmologist is very helpful in the long-term care of the paralyzed eye. More permanent mechanisms of protection, including gold weights and tarsal springs, may be utilized depending on the expected long-term facial function outcome.

Glossopharyngeal and vagus nerve injuries may result in significant swallowing dysfunction. This disability is magnified if these injuries occur in synchrony. Swallowing rehabilitation with a speech therapist is mandatory. If significant aspiration and dysphonia are present, thyroplasty and gastrostomy are considered. Thyroplasty helps to improve not only the patient's voice, but also pulmonary toilet. Thyroplasty is performed in the early postoperative period in an attempt to avoid a gastrostomy. Although once avoided, early gastrostomy is now encouraged to maximize the nutrition of the postsurgical patient, and may be removed when oral alimentation is sufficient.

◆ Conclusion

Great advances have been made in the development of modern neurotologic surgery. Current surgical and medical management techniques have significantly reduced the morbidity and mortality of neurotologic surgery. An understanding of the potential complications of surgery facilitates the appropriate evaluation and counseling of the preoperative patient and helps to reduce the incidence of perioperative complications.

Suggested Readings

Brackmann DE, Rodgers GK. Management of postoperative cerebrospinal fluid leaks. In: Brackmann DE, ed. Otologic Surgery. Philadelphia: WB Saunders, 2001:604-609

Briggs RJ, Luxford WM, Atkins JS Jr, Hitselberger WE. Translabyrinthine removal of large acoustic neuromas. Neurosurgery 1994;34:785–790, discussion 790–791

Friedman RA, Cullen RD, Ulis J, Brackmann DE. Management of cerebrospinal fluid leaks after acoustic tumor removal. Neurosurgery 2007;61(3, Suppl)35–39, discussion 39–40

Rodgers GK, Luxford WM. Factors affecting the development of cerebrospinal fluid leak and meningitis after translabyrinthine acoustic tumor surgery. Laryngoscope 1993;103:959–962

Slattery WH III, Francis S, House KC. Perioperative morbidity of acoustic neuroma surgery. Otol Neurotol 2001;22:895–902

16

Auditory Brainstem Implants

Jose N. Fayad, William M. Luxford, Derald E. Brackmann, and William E. Hitselberger

◆ Overview

In 1979, William F. House and William E. Hitselberger implanted a pair of electrodes into the cochlear nucleus of a human volunteer with neurofibromatosis type 2 (NF2) during a surgical procedure to remove a second side acoustic neuroma. Since then, more than 200 patients at our institution have undergone implantation with auditory brainstem implants (ABIs). Stimulation of the electrodes produces auditory sensation in most patients (90%), with results similar to those for a single-channel cochlear implant. More recently, a combination of a surface electrode and a penetrating electrode has been used, with the goal of taking advantage of cochlear nucleus complex tonotopic organization.

We developed the ABI for patients with NF2 to electrically stimulate the cochlear nucleus complex. Patients with NF2 usually have bilateral vestibular schwannomas (VSs), necessitating tumor removal, which often results in profound deafness. The ABI is introduced into the lateral recess of the fourth ventricle and placed over the area of the ventral and dorsal cochlear nuclei after tumor removal. The ABI is similar in design and function to multichannel cochlear implants (CIs), except for differences in the design of the stimulating electrode arrays. The programming of ABI devices, however, differs in several important aspects from CI programming. Multichannel CIs and ABIs were developed to capitalize on the frequency tuning of neurons in the human cochlea and cochlear nucleus complex, respectively. Cochlear implants, which electrically activate peripheral neural processes within the cochlea, are not an option for patients with NF2 because of their loss of integrity of the auditory nerve.

In multichannel CIs, the electrode is placed into the cochlea. Consistent placement of the electrode carrier and its depth of insertion are assured in normal cochleas. However, in ABI recipients, anatomic landmarks that are used in electrode array placement may be altered or obscured due to the presence of tumors, making electrode array placement more challenging. This chapter describes the surgical anatomy of the cochlear nucleus complex, and our experience and results with ABI placement in individuals with NF2.

◆ Patient Selection/Device and Results

With two exceptions, only patients with NF2 and bilateral acoustic neuromas have received the ABI at the House Clinic. In these patients, the goal is to restore some auditory function so that these individuals can continue to be a part of the hearing world and to improve their quality of life. The ABI is placed during removal of their first tumor even if they have hearing on the other side, which is usually the case. This approach allows patients to become familiar with the use of the device and prepares them for when all hearing is lost.

Table 16.1   Indications for Auditory Brainstem Implants
Classic indication:
Neurofibromatosis type 2; bilateral transverse temporal bone fractures
Emerging indications:
Cochlear nerve aplasia, cochlear ossification with limited benefit from cochlear implants

Other possible indications include bilateral transverse skull fractures and avulsion of both cochlear nerves. More recently, in Europe, the indications for the ABI have included cochlear nerve aplasia and severe cochlear malformations in children, and complete ossification of the cochlea or cochlear nerve disruption due to cochlear trauma in adults (**Table 16.1**).

The current surface electrode ABI consists of 21 electrodes embedded in a silicone carrier that is fixed to a fabric mesh, connected to an implantable internal receiver/stimulator (Cochlear Corp., Englewood, CO). It received Food and Drug Administration (FDA) approval for commercial use in 2000. The current investigational penetrating ABI (PABI) consists of two arrays, a 12-electrode surface array, plus a 10-electrode array with needle microelectrodes. The external equipment for both devices consists of an external transmitter coil held in place by magnetic tape placed on the scalp over the receiver/stimulator coil and connected to a sound processor and microphone, which contains the battery-operated power source. All of this is similar to a cochlear implant. As long as the magnet is removed from the implanted receiver/stimulator, follow-up serial magnetic resonance imaging (MRI) scans can be obtained, as the rest of the implanted hardware is nonferromagnetic.

The sound processing unit (speech processor) requires appropriate programming and must be fitted to the individual user. Programming speech processors involves psychophysical assessment of electrically induced auditory (and nonauditory) percepts including threshold, comfort level, and pitch. These measures are programmed into the processor and used to control the amplitude and the sequential patterns of stimulation. ABI recipients have variations in brainstem anatomy, electrode array placement, and tumor effects that require the use of more individualized stimulus patterns to code frequency cues, and manage any nonauditory sensations than is typical for cochlear implants. Special techniques and additional time is usually required to program ABI sound processors appropriately.

Initial stimulation is performed 1 to 2 months after the surgery. Any nonauditory sensations are reduced or, if possible, eliminated by altering the electrical parameters of stimulation (particularly pulse duration and reference ground electrode). Nonauditory sensations have included dizziness, sensation of vibration in the eye, throat sensations, and ipsilateral tingling sensations in the head or body. Stimulation for the surface ABI and the PABI differs in some respects. Because the PABI has two arrays (a surface and a penetrating array), the sound processor is configured with programs using each electrode array separately, and an additional program using a combination of electrodes from both arrays. Performance is assessed with each of these configurations, adding to the time necessary to manage these research patients.

To date, more than 500 patients have been implanted worldwide using the ABI. The safety of this device has been comparable to the safety of cochlear implants. About 92% of our patients have received auditory sensations from their ABIs, and 80% of those implanted are device users. Approximately 16% of patients have achieved limited open-set speech discrimination (at least 20% correct in sound only on the City University of New York [CUNY] Sentences Test). A few ABI recipients have scored in the vicinity of 50% or better in a sound-only condition on this test. The majority of the patients recognize some environmental sounds, and speech understanding ability is enhanced an average of 30% when ABI sound is added to lipreading cues. This enhancement has ranged up to as high as 70% improvement for some patients.

The PABI was developed in an effort to improve the precision of stimulation of brainstem auditory neurons, and is in the clinical trials phase under auspices of the FDA. Three PABI recipients implanted during phase I at House Research Institute (HRI) have been extensively tested over the past 2 years. The patients use their PABI devices daily, with benefit. Their performance has been stable, and speech perception as measured on the CUNY Sentences Test is improved an average of 30% in the sound plus lipreading condition (as compared with the lipreading only condition). PABI recipients report a wide range of pitch sensations on both penetrating and surface electrodes, which we believe enhances speech perception performance. The study will continue with implantation of up to 10 patients with the second-generation PABI.

◆ Surgical Anatomy

The cochlear nucleus complex (dorsal and ventral cochlear nuclei) lies in the lateral recess of the fourth ventricle. It is partially obscured by the cerebellar peduncles. A surface electrode introduced in the lateral recess crossing the tinea choroidea will stimulate viable cochlear nuclei.

Recently Abe and Rhoton described in detail the microsurgical anatomy of the cochlear nuclei. The vestibulocochlear nerve enters the brainstem slightly rostral and ventral to the foramen of Luschka near the flocculus at the lateral end of the pontomedullary sulcus. The facial nerve arises ventromedial to the vestibulocochlear nerve in the lateral part of the pontomedullary sulcus. The average distance between the center of the facial and cochlear nerves at their junction with the brainstem is 3.8 mm. The glossopharyngeal and vagus nerves arise caudal to the facial nerve. The average distance between the centers of the junction of the cochlear and glossopharyngeal nerves with the brainstem is 6.4 mm and between the facial and glossopharyngeal nerves is 6.3 mm.

The foramen of Luschka, the open end of the lateral recess of the fourth ventricle, is located slightly dorsal and caudal to the junction of the vestibulocochlear nerve with the brainstem, dorsal to the junction of the glossopharyngeal nerve with the brainstem, and ventral and caudal to the flocculus. The lateral recess is a narrow, curved pouch formed by the union of the roof and the floor of the fourth ventricle. The caudal wall of the recess is formed by the tela choroidea that stretches upward from the narrow ridge, called the taenia, along the lower edge of the fourth ventricle and lateral recess. The choroid plexus arises in and attaches to the inner surface of the tela. The lateral recess and the foramen of Luschka open into the medial part of the inferior limb of the cerebellopontine angle. The flocculus projects into the cerebellopontine angle at the rostral edge of the foramen of Luschka at the junction of the cerebellopontine and cerebellomedullary fissures. The choroid plexus extends through the lateral recess and the foramen of Luschka into the cerebellopontine angle and often sits on the posterior margin of the glossopharyngeal nerve.

The dorsal and ventral cochlear nuclei are positioned in the lateral recess near the foramen of Luschka. The dorsal cochlear nucleus produces a smooth prominence, the auditory tubercle, on the dorsal surface of the inferior cerebellar peduncle in the upper part of the floor of the lateral recess. The medial edge of the dorsal cochlea nucleus is located just lateral to the vestibular area. The ventral cochlear nucleus is positioned between the junction of the vestibulocochlear nerve with the brainstem and the lateral edge of the dorsal cochlear nucleus. The ventral cochlear nucleus does not produce a discrete prominence on the surface of the brainstem as does the dorsal cochlear nucleus, whose position is marked by the auditory tubercle. The ventral cochlear nucleus is often partially hidden by the rhomboid lip, choroid plexus, and flocculus protruding from the foramen of Luschka. The ventral cochlear nucleus has two parts, cisternal and ventricular, which are separated by the edge of the small ridge or taenia. The ventral cochlear nucleus commonly lies partially inside the foramen of Luschka within the lateral recess and partially outside the foramen within the cerebellopontine angle cistern with the taenia of the rhomboid lip crossing its lateral surface. Terr and Edgerton also noted that the attachment of the taenia along the rhomboid lip often crosses the lateral surface of the ventral cochlear nucleus. The vestibulocochlear nerve pursues a medial, posterior, and caudal course from the internal acoustic meatus to the brainstem. The cochlear nuclei are oriented in a more posterior direction than the vestibulocochlear nerve, thus creating an angle at the junction of the dorsal surface of the nerve and long axis of the cochlear nucleus that averages 138 degrees.

◆ Surgical Technique

We administer preoperative antibiotics and continue them for 24 hours postoperatively. Intraoperative furosemide and mannitol are given to allow gentle easier cerebellar retraction, if needed. We administer dexamethasone intravenously during the procedure and continue this for 24 hours postoperatively. Long-acting muscle relaxants are avoided during surgery so as not to interfere with facial nerve monitoring.

At the House Clinic we have exclusively used the translabyrinthine approach for placement of the ABI. More recently, we have been using a C-shaped incision that extends just 1 cm above the pinna (**Fig. 16.1**). It allows the placement of the internal receiver and magnet under the scalp. It is important that the incision not directly cross the area of the receiver/stimulator.

The translabyrinthine approach provides direct access to the cochlear nuclei. The jugular bulb is skeletonized to provide the widest access to this area. Anatomic land-

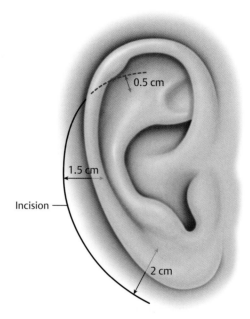

Fig. 16.1 C-shaped incision currently used for placement of an auditory brainstem implant (ABI).

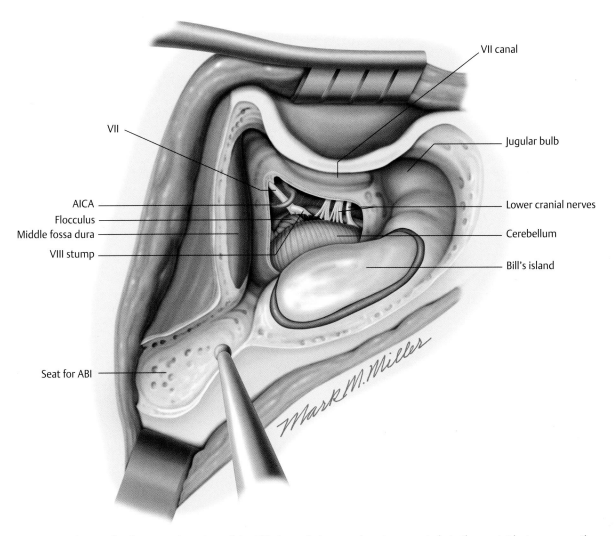

VII canal

VII

Jugular bulb

AICA

Flocculus

Middle fossa dura

VIII stump

Lower cranial nerves

Cerebellum

Bill's island

Seat for ABI

Mark M. Miller

Fig. 16.2 The seat for the internal receiver of the ABI electrode is created posterosuperiorly to the mastoidectomy, once the tumor is removed through the translabyrinthine approach. The stump of cranial nerve VIII is shown. AICA, anterior inferior cerebellar artery.

marks used for placement include the stump of cranial nerve VIII, the origin of the glossopharyngeal nerve from the brainstem, the facial nerve, and the tinea choroidea, as well as the mouth of the lateral recess where all of these structures converge (**Figs. 16.2, 16.3, and 16.4**). The two features used by the neurosurgeon in identifying the lateral recess are its relationship to cranial nerve IX and the position of the jugular bulb. The entrance to the lateral recess is directly above the origin of the glossopharyngeal nerve at the brainstem. In the surgical setting, where there is almost always distortion of the brainstem from the tumor, the lateral recess is superior to cranial nerve IX, which is generally in a fixed anatomic position. Going from there, we can get to the lateral recess in almost every case. The jugular bulb is important because its position may vary. Indeed, with a contracted mastoid and a high jugular bulb, the exposure may be more difficult, although it should not be an impediment to placement of the ABI electrode. The key is to have good exposure of the jugular bulb, which will augment the exposure of the lateral recess (see Technical Pearls, below).

Location of the ventral cochlear nucleus, the main target for placement of the ABI, can be problematic. Anatomic placement is confirmed using electrophysiologic mon-

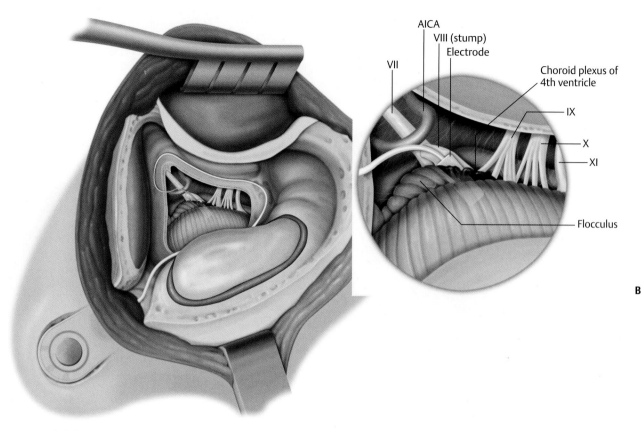

Fig. 16.3 **(A)** The internal receiver is in place under the periosteum posterosuperiorly. The wires cross through the craniotomy to reach the cerebellopontine angle. **(B)** The electrode is placed over the cochlear nucleus, in the lateral recess of the fourth ventricle. AICA, anterior inferior cerebellar artery.

itoring. Electrically evoked auditory brainstem responses are elicited by stimulation of the nucleus, and the position of the ABI electrode is optimized using information derived from electrophysiologic monitoring, with the help of an experienced auditory physiologist. Cranial nerve IX should be tamponaded away from the electrode plate to avoid any cardiac arrhythmias during placement. In addition to facial nerve monitoring, the lower cranial nerves are also monitored to avoid side effects and nonauditory sensations. Once the optimal position is determined, Teflon felt is used to secure the electrode in the lateral recess of the fourth ventricle. The internal receiver is fixed to the skull in a posterosuperior position to the mastoid defect; a seat is created in the bone to lower the profile of the internal receiver/stimulator, which is stabilized using nonresorbable sutures to the skull.

Others have used the retrosigmoid approach to implant the cochlear nucleus complex with similar success and results.

In the case of the PABI, after establishing of the landmarks and identification of the cochlear nuclei, the penetrating electrode is placed first into the ventral portion of the nucleus, which is then followed by placement of the surface electrode as in a regular ABI surgery.

Implantation is easier when the landmarks are preserved and the surface anatomy is normal, as is the case in the newest indications for the ABI: cochlear nerve aplasia and severe cochlear malformations in children, and complete ossification of the cochlea in adults.

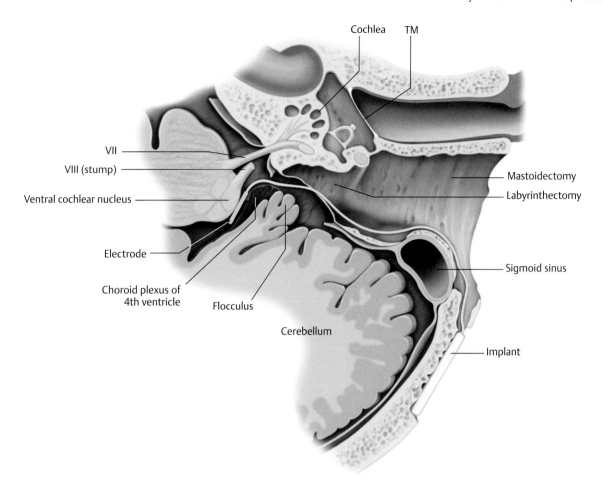

Fig. 16.4 Rendering of a horizontal cut showing the electrode in the lateral recess of the fourth ventricle against the ventral cochlear nucleus. TM, tympanic membrane.

◆ **Technical Pearls**

- The origin of cranial nerve IX at the brainstem will guide you to the lateral recess of the fourth ventricle.
- Follow the stump of cranial nerve VIII to the foramen of Luschka.
- Identify the choroid plexus at the mouth of the recess.
- Open the mouth of the recess and resect the choroid plexus if needed.
- Identify the tinea choroidea; it bisects the ventral cochlear nucleus.
- Follow the cochlear nuclear complex into the lateral recess of the fourth ventricle. The complex curves posterosuperiorly.
- Tuck the surface electrode under the inferior cerebellar peduncle and over the complex. Electrical stimulation confirms the location of the electrode.
- The penetrating electrode is implanted into the ventral cochlear nucleus.

◆ **Conclusion**

The ABI is introduced using a translabyrinthine approach into the lateral recess of the fourth ventricle and placed over the area of the ventral and dorsal cochlear nuclei after vestibular schwannoma removal. More than 200 patients have been implanted using the ABI at HEI, more than 500 worldwide. The safety of the stimulation of the cochlear nuclei using this device has been established. Most patients perceive useful auditory sensations and improve their communication abilities over lipreading only. A smaller number achieve substantial speech discrimination using only ABI sound. The majority of ABI recipients typically enjoys using the device regularly and finds it improves their quality of life.

Suggested Readings

Brackmann DE, Hitselberger WE, Nelson RA, et al. Auditory brainstem implant: I. Issues in surgical implantation. Otolaryngol Head Neck Surg 1993;108:624–633

Colletti V, Shannon RV, Carner M, Veronese S, Colletti L. Complications in auditory brainstem implant surgery in adults and children. Otol Neurotol 2010;31:558–564

Otto SR, House WF, Brackmann DE, Hitselberger WE, Nelson RA. Auditory brain stem implant: effect of tumor size and preoperative hearing level on function. Ann Otol Rhinol Laryngol 1990;99(10 Pt 1): 789–790

Sennaroglu L, Colletti V, Manrique M, et al. Auditory brainstem implantation in children and non-neurofibromatosis type 2 patients: a consensus statement. Otol Neurotol 2011;32:187–191

Shannon RV, Fayad J, Moore J, et al. Auditory brainstem implant: II. Postsurgical issues and performance. Otolaryngol Head Neck Surg 1993;108:634–642

Shannon RV, Otto SR. Psychophysical measures from electrical stimulation of the human cochlear nucleus. Hear Res 1990;47:159–168

17

The Fine Points of Posterior Fossa Surgery

William E. Hitselberger, Marc S. Schwartz,
and Rick A. Friedman

This final chapter enumerates the surgical techniques that we have developed to facilitate operative exposure, preservation of the facial nerve, preservation of the cochlear nerve, and avoidance of injury to adjacent neurologic structures, such as the brainstem and regional cranial nerves. We discuss the following operations: the suboccipital retrolabyrinthine craniotomy with vestibular nerve section, the middle fossa craniotomy, and the suboccipital translabyrinthine craniotomy.

◆ The Suboccipital Retrolabyrinthine Craniotomy with Vestibular Nerve Section

The indications for this procedure are refractory Meniere's disease or other pathology involving the vestibular nerves. It can be performed in association with an endolymphatic shunting procedure.

The procedure is performed with the patient in a supine position with the head turned away from the involved side. Head tongs are not necessary. If the neck is stiff and the degree of rotation is limited, the operating table itself can be rotated to compensate. The skin incision should be at least a fingerbreadth behind and parallel to the helix of the involved ear (**Fig. 17.1**). If the incision is too far forward in the auricular crease, the necessary bony dissection beneath the skin will be virtually impossible.

One of the key considerations in this operation, and in fact all operations through the temporal bone, is adequate exposure—the sine qua non of all temporal bone surgery. The skin is reflected and held in place with retractors exposing the underlying mastoid and subocciput. A complete mastoidectomy is then performed.

Bones should be completely removed over the sigmoid sinus so it can be easily decompressed. At least a centimeter of bone should be removed from the suboccipital area posterior to the sinus (**Fig. 17.2**). This is as critical (if not more so) than for the suboccipital translabyrinthine approach. If this is not done completely, a bothersome bony ridge will prevent adequate exposure in the cerebellopontine angle after the dura has been opened. Bone should be removed over the dura overlying the temporal lobe. It is far better and safer to make sure the bony exposure is adequate before opening the dura. To complete the bony dissection, bone should be removed medial to the posterior semicircular canal as far anteriorly as possible (**Fig. 17.2**). If the posterior semicircular canal is laterally placed, dissection can be performed almost to the internal auditory canal. One of the errors in the performance of this operation is inadequate bone removal. The importance of bone removal as described above cannot be overemphasized. If it is done properly, the procedure flows smoothly. If it is

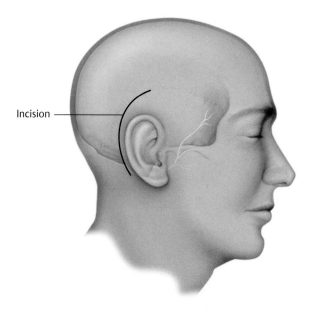

Fig. 17.1   Postauricular incision.

inadequate, it is impossible to clearly delineate cranial nerve VIII in the cerebellopontine angle.

The dural opening is squarely shaped with one limb inferior to the superior petrosal sinus and the other limb anterior to the sigmoid sinus (**Fig. 17.3**). The underlying cerebellum relaxes after removal of spinal fluid from the cisterna lateralis. Gentle pressure on the cerebellum using only a suction tip, with or without a cottonoid strip, will usually suffice to open the cistern. Once the cerebellopontine angle has been exposed, it is important to recognize the position and the relationships of cranial

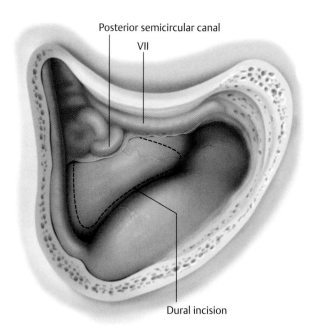

Fig. 17.2   Retrolabyrinthine posterior fossa and sigmoid sinus decompression.

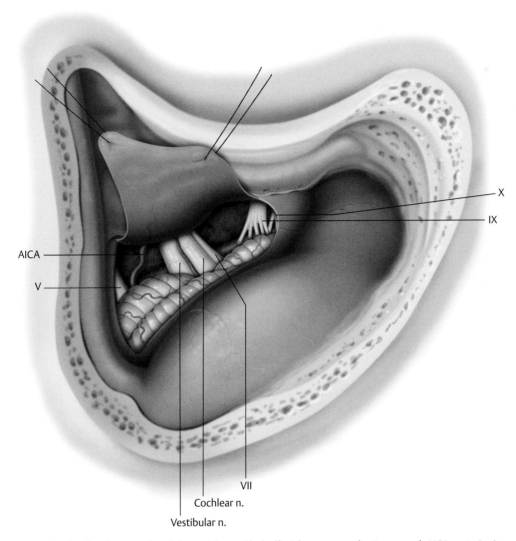

Fig. 17.3 The dura is opened and the cochleovestibular/facial nerve complex is exposed. AICA, anterior inferior cerebellar artery.

nerves VII and VIII. Occasionally they will be obscured by a small lobe of cerebellum. The cerebellum can sometimes be herniated into the porus of the internal auditory canal. This lobe of cerebellum should be carefully dissected free from the internal auditory canal. Then the plane between the cerebellum and the nerves can be cleanly developed.

The vestibular division of the cochlear nerve lies superior to the cochlear division in the cerebellopontine angle (**Fig. 17.3**). This is because of the rotation of cranial nerve VIII that occurs after it exits the internal auditory canal. The facial nerve usually lies anterior to cranial nerve VIII but occasionally will be superiorly placed, being very close to the vestibular division. It is extremely important to ascertain the position of the facial nerve with the facial nerve monitor. A small sharp hook can then be used to separate the fibers of the vestibular division from the cochlear division. This dissection is done on the superior aspect of cranial nerve VIII in an anterior to posterior direction. This method of dissection is utilized because of the kidney-bean shape of cranial nerve VIII in cross section. A glistening plane is usually visible between the vestibular and cochlear divisions when the section is complete (**Fig. 17.4**).

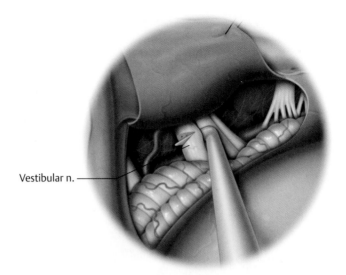

Vestibular n.

Fig. 17.4 Using a hook, the vestibular nerve is separated from the cochlear nerve and cut.

After completion of the section, the dura is sutured. The cavity is filled with abdominal fat and then covered with titanium mesh, which is fixed to the underlying bone with metallic screws.

◆ Suboccipital Translabyrinthine Craniotomy

The suboccipital translabyrinthine craniotomy is an extension of the suboccipital retrolabyrinthine craniotomy as described above. The additional dissection in this operation entails a complete labyrinthectomy, exposure of the internal auditory canal, and the labyrinthine portion of the facial nerve. This will assist in the retraction necessary for the further exposure needed in this procedure (**Figs. 17.5, 17.6, 17.7, and 17.8**). The dura is opened over the posterior fossa and the internal auditory canal (**Fig. 17.9**). The cut dural edges are tented up superiorly and inferiorly using 4-0 suture.

In the situation where there is a large underlying tumor, it is extremely important to decompress the cisterna lateralis of spinal fluid. This can be done either by retraction of the cerebellum using cottonoid strips and a suction device or removal of a portion of the interior of the tumor. These maneuvers usually open up the cisterna lateralis and release the spinal fluid. After this has been accomplished, the intracranial pressure will be relaxed and exposure in the cerebellopontine angle will be facilitated.

If the tumor is small, facial nerve dissection starts at the end of the internal auditory canal. Previously the labyrinthine portion of the facial nerve has been identified (**Fig. 17.10**). Starting from this known identifiable position at the lateral extent of the internal auditory canal, facial nerve dissection can begin. Cranial nerve VIII is cut laterally and all tumor is removed from the fundus of the internal auditory canal. The establishment of a plane between the facial nerve and the tumor at the lateral extent of the internal auditory canal is extremely important. The dissection in this plane can be developed down to the origin of the facial nerve at the brainstem. This in effect facilitates the total removal of the tumor. Care must be taken to avoid stretching of the facial nerve with small tumors that have not been already stretched over time with tumor growth. This is critical.

The dissection of a large tumor is of course much more difficult. The course of the facial nerve over the dome of the tumor is variable and must be considered. The

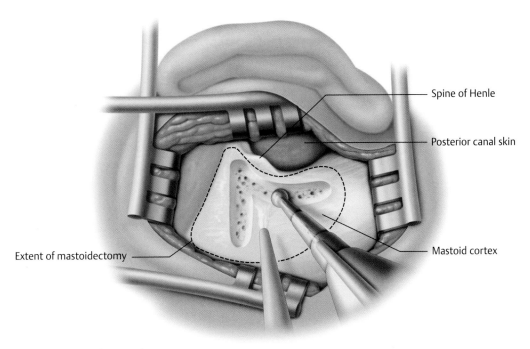

Fig. 17.5 Cortical mastoidectomy.

Spine of Henle

Posterior canal skin

Mastoid cortex

Extent of mastoidectomy

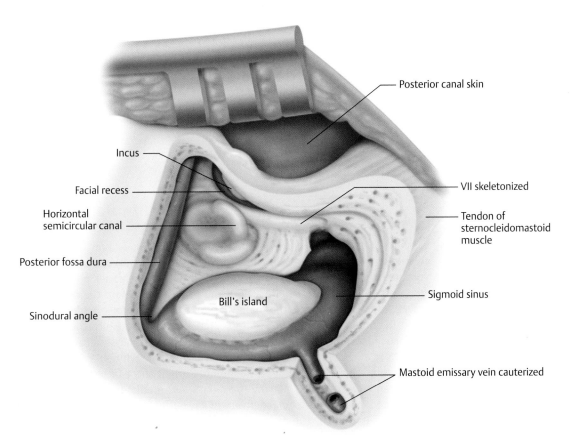

Fig. 17.6 Complete mastoidectomy.

Posterior canal skin

Incus

Facial recess

Horizontal
semicircular canal

Posterior fossa dura

Bill's island

Sinodural angle

VII skeletonized

Tendon of
sternocleidomastoid
muscle

Sigmoid sinus

Mastoid emissary vein cauterized

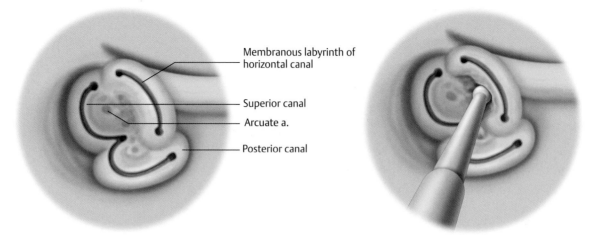

A   B

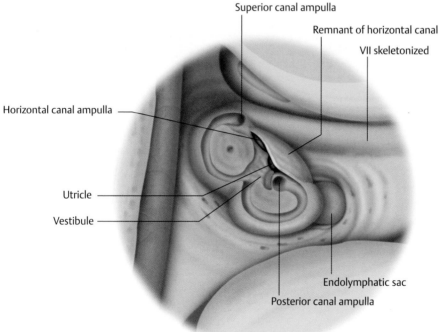

C

Membranous labyrinth of horizontal canal

Superior canal

Arcuate a.

Posterior canal

Superior canal ampulla

Remnant of horizontal canal

VII skeletonized

Horizontal canal ampulla

Utricle

Vestibule

Endolymphatic sac

Posterior canal ampulla

Fig. 17.7   (A–C) Labyrinthectomy.

dissections of tumors with an anteriorly placed facial nerve are in general less complicated than for a superiorly placed facial nerve. The exact position of the facial nerve should be ascertained early in the procedure. Before the facial nerve can be saved and dissected free, the main mass of the tumor must be debulked and delivered. In our hands this can be accomplished either with the ultrasonic aspirator or the Urban rotary dissector. The tumor is usually crushed over small areas with a cupped forceps to allow better uptake with either of these instruments. Once the main mass of the tumor has been removed, the point of origin of the facial nerve from the brainstem can be ascertained. Having the lateral and medial portions of the facial nerve delineated facilitates the final delivery of the nerve from the tumor. Dissection of the facial nerve from the tumor is performed with sharp dissection, avoiding tension or pulling on the facial nerve as much as possible. This part of the dissection can be extremely difficult. Occasionally a small scrap of tumor may be left on the facial nerve if it is apparent that removing it will result in loss of continuity of the nerve.

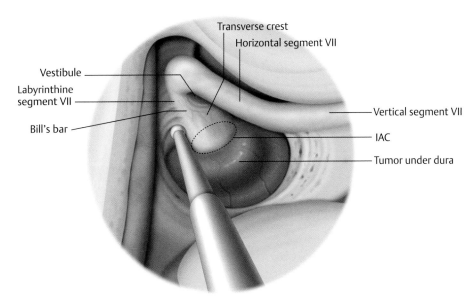

Fig. 17.8   Facial nerve identification. IAC, internal auditory canal.

Arterial dissection is as important, if not more so, than the facial nerve dissection. If a major artery is interrupted, injury to the adjacent brainstem can occur with subsequent serious neurologic sequelae. Arterial dissection should proceed from the smaller branches down toward the main trunk, rather than trying to dissect the main trunk itself. The smaller radicals of the artery can be dissected free from the tumor without injury, but if the main trunk is damaged a brainstem infarct can result.

Closure of the dura is important. The authors use a continuous 4-0 silk suture to approximate the edges of the dura (**Fig. 17.11**). The mastoid cavity is filled with

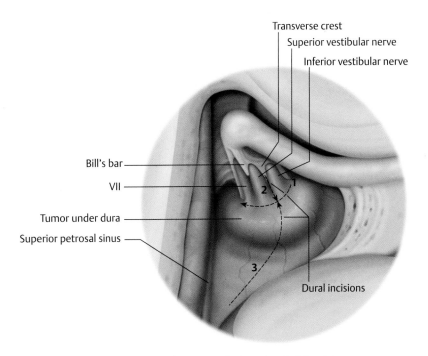

Fig. 17.9   Internal auditory canal nerves in the lateral end of the IAC.

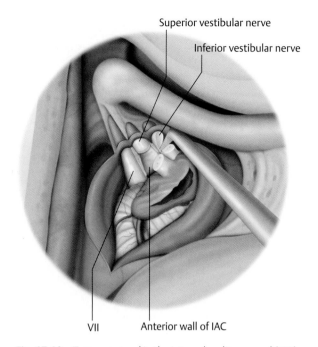

Fig. 17.10 Tumor removal in the internal auditory canal (IAC).

abdominal fat. The middle ear is obliterated with muscle and Surgicel. The aditus of the middle ear can be covered with temporalis fascia. Titanium mesh is placed over the cavity and secured with metallic screws to the surrounding bone as in the retro-labyrinthine approach (**Fig. 17.12**).

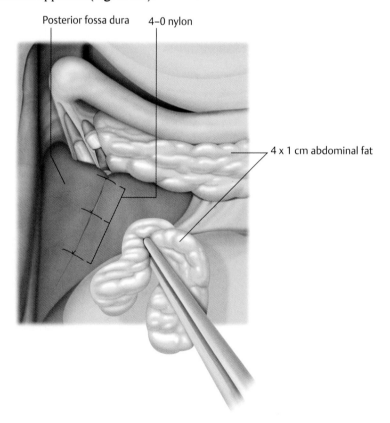

Fig. 17.11 Dural closure and fat packing.

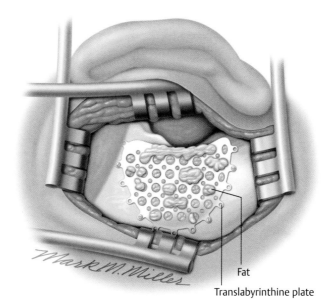

Fat

Translabyrinthine plate

Fig. 17.12   Cranioplasty.

◆ Middle Fossa Craniotomy

This procedure is used for tumors confined to the internal auditory canal or protruding slightly into the posterior fossa. The upper limit of tumor size for this approach is usually about 1 cm in maximal diameter in the cerebellopontine angle in a patient with good hearing. The middle fossa approach is performed with the patient supine and the head turned away from the involved side. An adequate skin shave over the involved side is important. The incision runs from the tragus anteriorly and then superiorly curving around the helix of the ear and then swinging anteriorly to end behind the hair line—the so-called question-mark incision (**Fig. 17.13**). The underlying muscle layer is swung forward with the skin. Both of these layers are fixed to the drapes. A small remnant of temporalis muscle is left intact at the base of the incision above the zygomatic arch (**Fig. 17.14**).

The bone flap measures 5 cm along the base and 6 cm along the inferosuperior aspect. It is important that the base of the bone flap be approximately three quarters anterior to the external auditory canal and one quarter posterior (**Fig. 17.15**). If the base of the bone flap is positioned too far posteriorly, exposure of the internal auditory canal will be extremely difficult. The dura is dissected from the middle fossa floor down to the petrous ridge. It is usually not necessary to expose the middle meningeal artery at the foramen spinosum.

The placement of the retractor over the dura overlying the temporal lobe is extremely important. Retraction of the dura allows exposure of the internal auditory canal from above. The blades should be placed over the most medial limit of the petrous ridge, that is, the "true" petrous ridge. This occasionally can be difficult to do, but if done properly it augments the exposure of the internal auditory canal.

The internal auditory canal is usually in the trough lying anterior to the arcuate eminence. The arcuate eminence overlies the region of the superior semicircular canal and generally can be easily seen. The internal auditory canal is usually found in the middle of the angle subtended by the arcuate eminence and the greater superficial petrosal nerve, which should be exposed (**Fig. 17.16**). Further identification of the internal auditory canal is obtained by observing the small protrusion of the petrous ridge directly over the internal auditory canal.

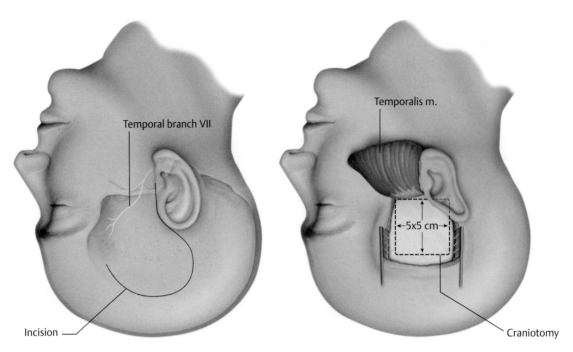

Fig. 17.13 Preauricular/temporal scalp incision. Note position of frontal branch of cranial nerve VII.

Fig. 17.14 Skin flap and temporalis muscle reflected, demonstrating the outline of the temporal craniotomy.

The exposure of the internal auditory canal should be approximately 270 degrees circumference at the porus and 135 degrees at the lateral extent of the canal. Exposure at the lateral end of the canal may be difficult because of the danger of rupture into the cochlea or the ampulla of the superior semicircular canal. However, this exposure is critical especially if the tumor arises from the inferior vestibular nerve and

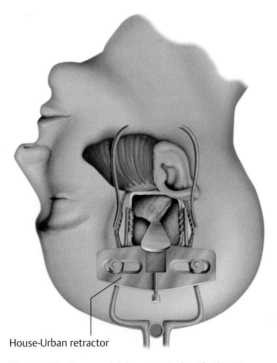

Fig. 17.15 Temporal lobe retracted with the House-Urban retractor place in the true petrous ridge after elevation of the superior petrosal sinus within the dura.

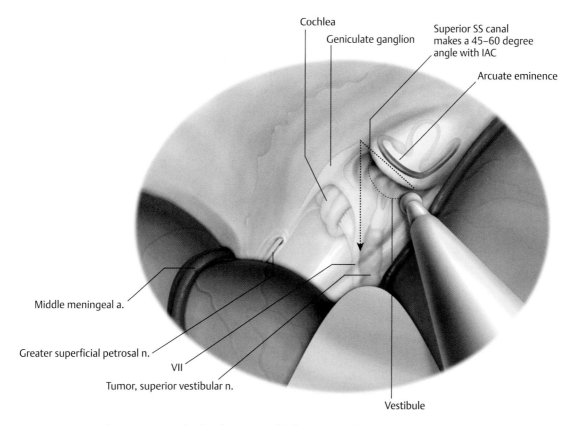

Cochlea

Geniculate ganglion

Superior SS canal
makes a 45–60 degree
angle with IAC

Arcuate eminence

Middle meningeal a.

Greater superficial petrosal n.

VII

Tumor, superior vestibular n.

Vestibule

Fig. 17.16 Critical microanatomic landmarks. Diamond ball no greater than 2.0 mm can be safely used to remove the bone of the lateral interior auditory canal. SS, semicircular.

is inferior to the transverse crest. The surgeon should be able to palpate the end of the internal auditory canal with a 1-mm blunt hook if the exposure has been adequate.

The dura is opened over the posterior aspect of the internal auditory canal (**Fig. 17.17**). The incision extends into the posterior fossa. The facial nerve will usually (but not always) be found in the anterior superior quadrant of the internal auditory canal

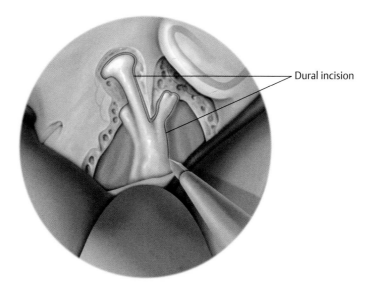

Dural incision

Fig. 17.17 The posterior dural incision over the tumor is reflected anteriorly.

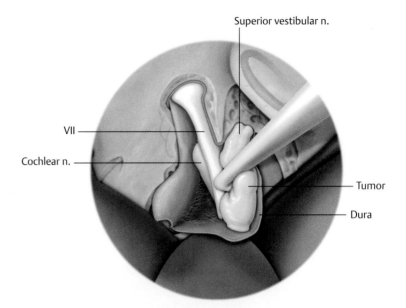

Fig. 17.18   The facial nerve is fully delineated and dissected free from the tumor prior to tumor removal.

(**Fig. 17.18**). The facial nerve should be separated from the tumor, going from lateral to medial in the internal auditory canal using sharp and blunt dissection. If the tumor arises from the inferior vestibular nerve, the superior vestibular nerve can be sectioned. This will allow exposure of the medial extent of the tumor. Whenever possible, tumor dissection should be from medial to lateral (as opposed to facial nerve dissection) to avoid avulsion of the delicate cochlear nerve fibers at the modiolus. This can occur if the dissection is initiated laterally. It is important to free all attachment of the tumor to the dura and from the vestibular nerve of origin using sharp hooked instruments. If exposure is adequate, the tumor can be delivered posteriorly out of the internal auditory canal (**Figs. 17.18 and 17.19**). With bulky tumors having

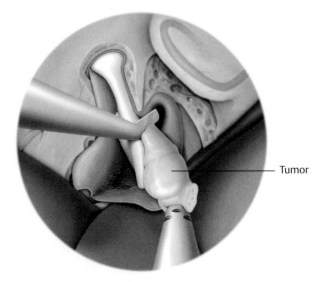

Fig. 17.19   Tumor is being removed after freeing it medially. Tumor is dissected from medial to lateral with extreme care in the region of the fundus beneath the transverse crest.

extension into the cerebellopontine angle, tumors can be debulked first before attempting to remove them.

The closure is extremely important. Occasionally there will be exposed air cells over the epitympanum and along the petrous ridge. These air cells should be sealed with bone wax. Fat should be placed in the opening in the dura over the internal auditory canal. The wound bed itself is covered with temporalis fascia. The bone flap is fixed to the surrounding calvaria with small titanium plates and screws to preserve the contour of the skull.

◆ Technical Pearls

- Extensive retrosigmoid bony decompression is important to allow for compression of the sinus and access along the petrous ridge.
- The vestibular portion of the nerve is superiorly oriented in the cerebellopontine angle.
- Identification of the plane between the vestibular and cochlear portions is most readily accomplished from anterior to posterior by using a nerve hook over the superior edge of the nerve.

◆ Conclusion

Transtemporal routes provide ideal access to the cerebellopontine angle and internal auditory canal. This is true whether inner ear structures are preserved, as with the retrolabyrinthine and middle fossa exposures, or sacrificed, as with the translabyrinthine exposure. Retraction of cerebellum can be almost entirely avoided, and temporal retraction is performed entirely extradurally. Adequate bony decompression, however, is critical.

Suggested Readings
Brackmann DE, House JR III, Hitselberger WE. Technical modifications to the middle fossa craniotomy approach in removal of acoustic neuromas. Am J Otol 1994;15:614–619
Hitselberger WE. Translabyrinthine approach to acoustic tumors. Am J Otol 1993;14:7–8 No abstract available.
Nguyen CD, Brackmann DE, Crane RT, Linthicum FH Jr, Hitselberger WE. Retrolabyrinthine vestibular nerve section: evaluation of technical modification in 143 cases. Am J Otol 1992;13:328–332

Index

Note: Page references followed by *f* indicate figures; page references followed by *t* indicate tables.

bacitracin irrigation in, 61
cerebrospinal fluid leak management in, 168*f*
closure of, 166
complications of, 65, 66*t*
cranioplasty in, 63–64, 63*f*
dural closure in, 62, 63*f*
facial nerve monitoring n, 49, 50*f*
incisions in, 49–51, 50*f*
internal auditory canal in, 56–57, 58*f*
intradural dissection in, 57–60, 58*f*
labyrinthectomy in, 53–55, 54*f*
limitations to, 67
mastoidectomy in, 51–53, 51*f*, 52*f*
mastoid emissary vein in, 53
middle ear and eustachian tube plugging in, 56
patient positioning for, 49
posterior fossa dissection in, 52–53, 52*f*
postoperative care following, 64
preparation for, 48–49
results of, 64–66
Transmastoid approach, *versus* retrosigmoid approach, 39
Transtentorial approach, combined with retrosigmoid approach, 38
Transverse sinus, 38–39
Trigeminal nerve. *See* Cranial nerve(s), V
Trigeminal neuralgia, microvascular cranial nerve decompression treatment for, 158, 160–161, 161*f*

Tympanic membrane, anatomy of, 120*f*

V
Vagus nerve. *See* Cranial nerve, X
Vascular lesions, far lateral approach to, 92
Vein of Labbé, 170–171
in combined petrosal approach, 88–89, 89*f*
in Fisch infratemporal fossa approach, 109, 113
in temporal bone reconstruction, 155
Vertebral artery
anatomy of, 93–94
in far lateral approach, 93–94, 94*t*, 101*f*, 104*f*, 105–106
in transcochlear approach, 76, 78*f*
Vertebrobasilar junction, in far lateral approach, 102–103, 105–106
Vertebrobasilar system, vascular disorders of, retrosigmoid approach to, 39*t*
Vestibular nerve
inferior, in translabyrinthine approach, 60, 60*f*
microvascular decompression of, 163
in middle cranial fossa approach, 24
schwannomas of
auditory brainstem implants for, 179–180
hearing preservation in, 29*t*

middle cranial fossa approach to, 19–30
translabyrinthine approach to, 47–66
in suboccipital retrolabyrinthine craniotomy, 183, 183*f*, 184*f*
superior, in translabyrinthine approach, 58*f*, 59–60, 60*f*
in temporal bone resection, 149*f*
Vestibule, in translabyrinthine approach, 54, 54*f*, 55*f*
Vestibulocochlear nerve. *See* Cranial nerve(s), VIII
Vocal cords, paralysis or paresis of, 94–95

W
Wound breakdown, temporal bone reconstruction-related, 156
Wound infections, postoperative, 170
preauricular infratemporal approach-related, 140

Z
Zygoma
exposure of, 3, 4*f*
in subtemporal approach, 14, 14*f*
Zygomatic arch
in Fisch infratemporal fossa approach, 127, 127*f*, 128*f*
in orbitozygomatic craniotomy, 1, 3, 4*f*, 5, 5*f*, 8
in preauricular infratemporal fossa approach, 135, 136f
in temporal bone resection, 153